FLAPS
DECISION MAKING
IN
CLINICAL PRACTICE

Springer
New York
Berlin
Heidelberg
Barcelona
Budapest
Hong Kong
London
Milan
Paris
Santa Clara
Singapore
Tokyo

FLAPS

DECISION MAKING
IN
CLINICAL PRACTICE

THE MEMBERS OF THE ONEIRO TRAVEL CLUB

L. FRANKLYN ELLIOTT

JAMES H. FRENCH, JR.

JAMES C. GROTTING

MCKAY MCKINNON

MICHAEL H. MOSES

RICHARD S. STAHL

BRYANT A. TOTH

VINCENT N. ZUBOWICZ

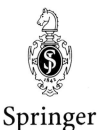

Springer

L. Franklyn Elliott, M.D., and the Members of the Oneiro Travel Club
975 Johnson Ferry Road, NE
Suite 500
Atlanta, GA 30342
USA

This project was conceived by Martin Dunitz Ltd., London.

The original artwork contained in this book was prepared by William M. Winn of the Scottish Rite Children's Medical Center of Atlanta, GA.

Library of Congress Cataloging-in-Publication Data
FLAPS : decision making in clinical practice / L. Franklyn Elliott . . .
  [et al.].
     p. cm.
  Includes bibliographical references and index.
  ISBN 0-387-94738-8 (hardcvr : alk. paper)
  1. Flaps (Surgery) 2. Surgery—Decision making. I. Elliott, L.
Franklyn.
  [DNLM: 1. Surgical Flaps. 2. Surgery, Plastic—methods. WO 610
F585 1997]
RD120.8.F53 1997
617.9'5—dc20
                                      96-23107

Printed on acid-free paper.

Production managed by Lesley Poliner; manufacturing supervised by Joe Quatela.
Typeset by Impressions Book and Journal Services, Inc., Madison, WI.
Printed and bound by Walsworth Publishing Co., Marceline, MO.
Printed in the United States of America.

9 8 7 6 5 4 3 2 1

ISBN 0-387-94738-8 Springer-Verlag New York Berlin Heidelberg SPIN 10534483

PREFACE

A textbook is a tool that has intentional purpose and use. Even when the same topic is covered, two books may have a completely different scope and focus. Depending upon the needs of the reader, one of the texts may be of great value while the other may be of little interest at all.

An author may choose to cover a certain range of material comprehensively, reviewing all that has been written about the subject as well as experienced firsthand. These encyclopedias are generally heavily referenced and authoritative. They may, however, lack focus. On the other hand, "how to do it" texts are intentionally pragmatic and useful. When they are the product of one or several authors, they may omit useful options because of the biases of the authors. Many times alternative philosophies or methodologies are ignored even when they may be commonly embraced.

The Oneiro travel club, after appreciable debate, decided to construct this text as a utilitarian manual on regional reconstructive problems. We felt that the collective wisdom of the authors, who are active practicing surgeons, could contribute a "real-life" look at surgical dilemmas. There is probably little that is revolutionary in this textbook. Rather, the emphasis is on a pragmatic look at regional reconstruction, the distillation and amalgamation of encyclopedic and "how I do it" approaches.

This collection should be controversial. The authors have agreed to be opinionated about their topics. By necessity, some workhorses will be ridden again and some sacred cows will be slain. But because the topics are covered by committee, even though the opening discussion is authored by individual writers, the emerging philosophies should be objective and thus useful.

This book is organized by anatomic region. The assignments were distributed to each author based on their familiarity with reconstruction in these regions. Each chapter consists of introductory text followed by a roundtable discussion of all the authors. The introductory text reflects the biases of each author tempered by the input of all the authors and the editorial process. If it stopped here, the book would be similar to many other texts that are assemblages of the writings of a number of authorities collected and edited by one or several individuals.

This text, however, includes and emphasizes the roundtable discussion that completes each chapter. It is here that controversies will be exposed and discussed. Some of these controversies may be nearly resolved by our group. Others will remain open to many approaches (which probably means there is no good solution). The roundtable discussion is a key ingredient to the uniqueness of the text and must be considered essential reading if the book is to provide the intended benefit.

What of the credibility of the authors? What do we have to say that others have not? The members of the Oneiro travel club are roughly the same age, about 10 years away from the completion of residency. Our training backgrounds are diverse, different residencies around the country reflecting differing strengths and philosophies. Similarly, our postgraduate professional lives have taken all of us to different geographic areas. Several of the members have pursued academic careers, some private practice, and some mixtures of both. All of us maintain a keen interest in the academic side of plastic surgery.

In short, we have been practicing long enough to gain a measure of experience in most areas of reconstruction. Better yet, there is no good reason for us to agree or disagree on fundamental problems of reconstruction other than by the coincidence of our collective experiences and observations. We have not evolved from one academic philosophy, nor have we migrated to one region, or fallen under the spell of one school of thought. It is hoped this translates into objectivity in the conclusions of this text.

If there is a "niche" to be filled by this book, it is for the reader who wants the opinion of experienced plastic surgeons who have no particular philosophy to espouse. Although each of us harbors strong opinions about the way certain reconstructive problems should be handled, the process of assembling this book submerges these opinions in the collective wisdom of the authors. We only hope that we are collectively wise enough to have created a book that will benefit the reader.

Vincent N. Zubowicz, M.D.

Contents

CONTRIBUTORS

Carl Colwell Askren, M.D.
Assistant Clincal Professor
UCSF-Fresno
Department of Surgery
6153 N. Thesta Avenue
Fresno, CA 93710

L. Franklyn Elliott, M.D.
Assistant Clinical Professor of Surgery
Emory University
Suite 500
975 Johnson Ferry Road, NE
Atlanta, GA 30342

Bryan G. Forley, M.D.
Attending Surgeon
Beth Israel Medical Center
Department of Plastic Surgery
5 East 82nd Street
New York, NY 10028

James Harold French, Jr., M.D.
Assistant Clinical Professor of Plastic Surgery
Georgetown University
Chief of Plastic Surgery, Fairfax Hospital
3299 Woodburn Road
Annandale, VA 22003

James C. Grotting, M.D., F.A.C.S.
Clinical Professor of Plastic Surgery
University of Alabama at Birmingham
Department of Surgery
Division of Plastic Surgery
McCollough, Grotting & Associates
Plastic Surgery Clinic, P.C.
1600 20th Street South
Birmingham, AL 35205

Gary S. Kopf, M.D.
Professor of Cardiac Surgery
Yale University of Medicine
333 Cedar Street
New Haven, CT 06510

McKay McKinnon, MD.
919 North Michigan Avenue
Suite #3100
Chicago, IL 60611

Michael H. Moses, M.D.
Clinical Assitant Professor of Surgery
Louisiana State University
Department of Surgery
1603 Second Street
New Orleans, LA 70130

Richard S. Stahl, M.D., M.B.A.
Associate Chief
Department of Surgery
Yale-New Haven Hospital
Clinical Professor of Surgery
Yale University School of Medicine
CB 228
20 York Street
New Haven, CT 06504

Bryant A. Toth, M.D.
Assistant Clinical Professor of Surgery
University of California, San Francisco
Attending Plastic Surgeon,
California Pacific Medical Center
2100 Webster Street, Suite #424
San Francisco, CA 94115

Vincent N. Zubowicz, M.D.
Clinical Professor of Plastic Surgery
Emory University Hospital
Department of Plastic Surgery
365 East Paces Ferry Road, NE
Atlanta, GA 30305

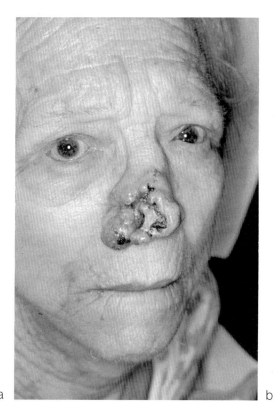

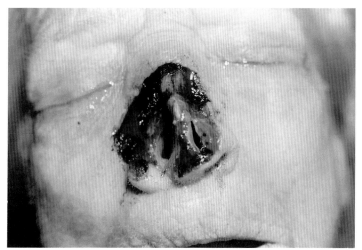

Figure 1.1. (a) Preoperative view of bulky basal cell carcinoma of the entire nasal tip. (b) Post-Mohs' defect of three-fourths of the nose, including a full-thickness defect of the lining and cartilage of the entire right nasal vestibule.

a

b

resultant amputation of two-thirds of the nose, including the entire tip. The patient was scheduled for immediate reconstruction on the day following the Mohs' surgery (Figure 1.1a, b).

THE SOLUTION

Reconstruction was performed under general anesthesia. Lining on the left side was provided by undermining and direct primary closure of the vestibular skin and mucosa laterally to the septal mucosa medially. The larger mucosal defect on the patient's right was closed with a pennant-shaped flap of buccal mucosa, based at the level of the right lateral maxillary incisor[1] and extending laterally in the labial-buccal sulcus (Figure 1.1c). The flap was tunneled through the soft tissues between the nose and the mouth and provided lining for the entire nasal tip unit. Cephalad to the flap, direct closure was achieved between the septal mucosa medially and the lateral nasal side-

ADAPTABLE NASAL RECONSTRUCTION WITH AN AXIAL FOREHEAD FLAP

MICHAEL H. MOSES

INTRODUCTION

Historically, the Indian method of nasal reconstruction with forehead flaps and Tagliacozzi's arm flap methods are two of the earliest described procedures in the specialty that was to become plastic surgery. Now, extensive nasal defects are more likely due to ablation from tumor than from trauma. But despite the miraculous advances in our field, complex nasal defects—large nasal surface areas missing with underlying structural and/or lining defects—remain one of the toughest challenges in modern plastic surgery.

THE PROBLEM

An 81-year-old woman presented with a basal cell carcinoma on the tip of her nose that had been ignored for 20 years. The tumor had largely destroyed her nasal tip, including much of both alae, a portion of the dorsum, and the anterior septum. It was fixed to the nasal lining. The patient was referred to the Mohs' dermatologist, who removed the tumor with a

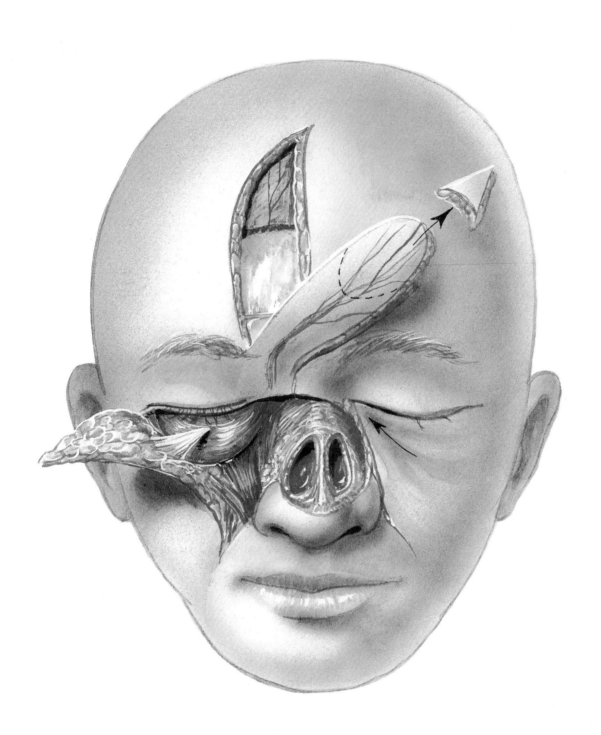

1

DECISION MAKING
IN
HEAD AND NECK
RECONSTRUCTION

(c) Pedicled buccal mucosal flap from the buccal sulcus to the nose to provide lining for the missing vestibule. (d) Final result, 2 weeks after division and inset of the forehead flap.

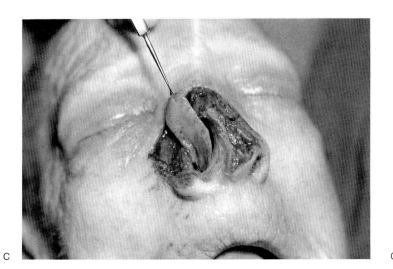

c

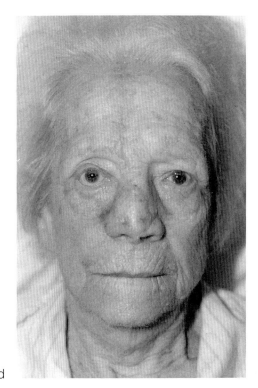

d

wall mucosa. Submucous cartilaginous resection of the residual septum was undertaken through existing mucosal incisions, and cartilage grafts were harvested to provide support for the middle third of the nose. The nasal tip skeletal support was reconstructed with conchal cartilage grafts.

External nasal cover was obtained with the combination of three flaps: a 4-cm-wide forehead flap based on the left supratrochlear artery, with two medial advancement flaps of both cheeks in the subcutaneous facelift plane with perialar crescenteric excisions to allow closure adjacent to the alae. Three weeks after the forehead flap was performed, the pedicle was divided and inset (Figure 1.1d).

Anatomy

The forehead flap is designed as an axial flap based on the supratrochlear neurovascular bundle. The supratrochlear vessels and nerve exit from the superomedial corner of the superior orbit. From the orbital rim, the artery courses directly cephalad, with very little deviation, for at least the first 8 cm above the orbit. The neurovascular bundle is consistent in this location in all patients operated upon, in anatomic atlases, and in anatomic dissections (Figure 1.2).

At the level of the orbit, the neurovascular bundle is just superficial to the frontal bone periosteum. At approximately 1 to 2 cm above the orbit, the artery runs at the level of the undersurface of the frontalis muscle. At approximately 5 to 7 cm above the orbits, the artery is superficial in the plane of the frontalis muscle. Where the frontalis muscle becomes aponeurotic more cephalad to this, the artery courses in the subcutaneous

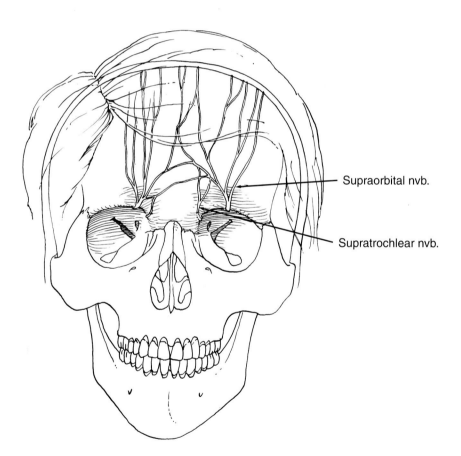

Supraorbital nvb.

Supratrochlear nvb.

Figure 1.2. Anatomic course of the supratrochlear neurovascular bundle. The supratrochlear artery and nerve exit from the superomedial corner of the orbit deep to the periosteum and extend directly cephalad in a predictable and constant manner.

tissue of the forehead deep to the dermis and superficial to the galea.

Because of this change in the layers of its axial vascular supply, the flap is designed with varying thickness over its length to include the artery but to minimize the thickness of the actual skin island to be transferred to the nose. Thus, the proximal 2 cm of the flap above the orbital rim is harvested in the subperiosteal plane. The next section of the flap, from 2 cm above the orbit to halfway through the desired skin island, is harvested in the subfrontalis or subgaleal plane. The cephalad, or distal, one-half of the proposed skin island is harvested as a skin-only random extension of the flap, with a minimum of subcutaneous fat (Figure 1.3).

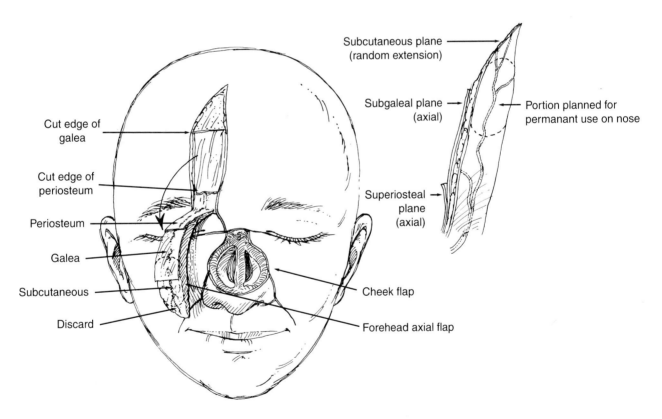

Figure 1.3. Three-layer "construction" of the axial forehead flap. The inferior 1.5 to 2 cm of the flap is subperiosteal. From there to the midpoint of the proposed skin island the flap is elevated in the subgaleal or subfrontalis muscle plane. The distal one-half of the skin island and the excision of the dog-ear are in the immediate subcutaneous plane.

TECHNIQUE

Forehead flap reconstructions may be performed under general anesthesia or under local anesthesia with intravenous sedation. A combination of bilateral supratrochlear and infraorbital nerve blocks with local infiltration for hemostasis will provide excellent regional anesthesia. All subsequent pedicle divisions and defatting procedures are easily done under local anesthesia with sedation.

Closure is undertaken from within outwards. First, lining defects are reconstructed. The general principle of lining reconstruction is to use "like for like": lining tissues should be reconstructed by similar lining tissues. Local advancement flaps of mucosa from within the nose, bipedicled intranasal lining flaps, or pedicled oral or nasal mucosal flaps are the three choices for lining deficits.[1,2]

Small lining defects can be closed primarily by undermining the adjacent lining. For slightly larger defects, a bipedicled flap of nasal lining based medially on the septum and laterally on the nasal sidewalls anterior to the turbinates can provide lining for the alae and lower third of the nose. Ideally, the raw space from the bipedicled flap will be beneath the nasal bones where it can reepithelialize secondarily without contracture of the reconstructed portion of the nose. For larger nasal lining defects, a nasal septal mucosal flap, as described by Burget,[2] has been utilized. For patients requiring even more extensive lining reconstructions, a large-pedicled, pennant-shaped buccal sulcus flap from the mouth[1] (as in the problem case; see Figure 1.4) can provide a large surface of vascularized, supple lining tissue. There must be adequate lining of the entire vestibule to avoid flap contracture from deficits of lining beneath the reconstructed tip.

Once internal airway lining has been accomplished, cartilaginous structural support is replaced as necessary. Cartilage grafts must be secured to adjacent remnants of secure structural support to provide an interlocking, self-supporting structure for the reconstructed portions of the nose. For small defects, septal cartilage can be harvested from within the nose by a submucosal technique. For larger structural needs, septal carti-

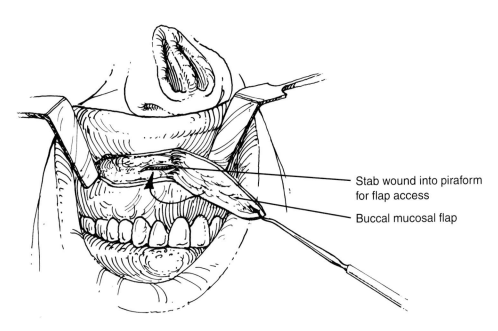

Stab wound into piraform
for flap access

Buccal mucosal flap

Figure 1.4. Pedicled buccal sulcus flaps may be passed from the mouth into the nasal defect to provide a large area of vascularized lining tissue. They should be based medially at the level of the lateral incisor and be harvested from buccal mucosa just above the labial-buccal sulcus.

lage can be combined with conchal cartilage. For reconstruction of the lower lateral cartilages, the convexity of the conchal cartilage is well suited to simulate the alar cartilage domes. In addition, cartilage grafts must also be placed along the nasal rim to buttress the rim downwards as a "batten," as described by Burget.[2,3,4] Septal or conchal cartilage may also be used to reconstruct structural defects of the upper lateral cartilages and/or nasal bones as well. Cartilage grafts should be securely fixed with sutures to resist the deformation that occurs with flap edema and its resolution.

The reconstructed alar cartilage should exactly match the contours of its opposite, whether it be reconstructed or native (see Photo 5a, 5b, 5c, and 6c). At the time of the construction of structural support, one must presume that the cover tissues will be exactly the same thickness as the remaining normal skin on the nose. Therefore, no allowance should be made in the cartilage reconstruction for additional skin thickness discrepancy.

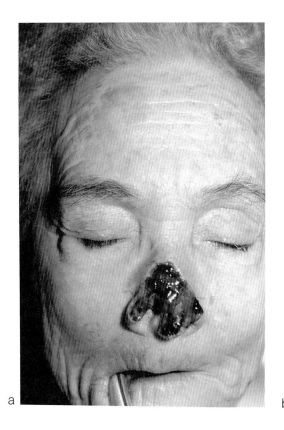

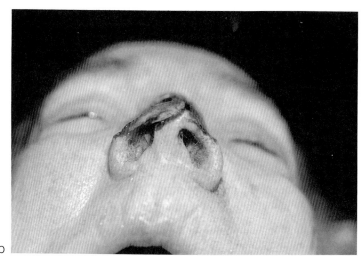

a

b

Figure 1.5. (a) Lower-half nasal defect with full-thickness defect of the right alar rim including cartilage and lining. (b) Basal view of the nose after lining reconstruction showing cartilage grafts to reconstruct the missing right alar cartilage.

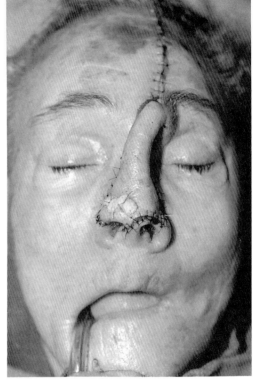

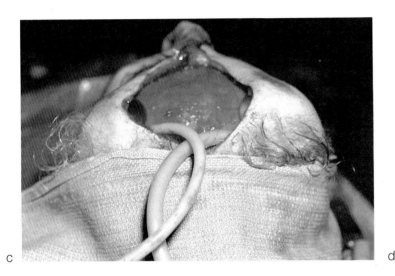

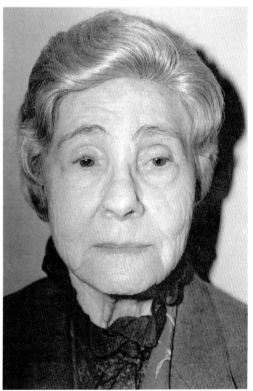

(c) Immediate intraoperative tissue expansion of the forehead to facilitate closure. (d) Intraoperative view after forehead flap cover showing symmetric tip projection and contour in a single stage. (e) Final postoperative result.

c

d

e

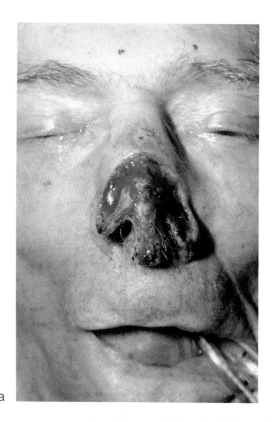

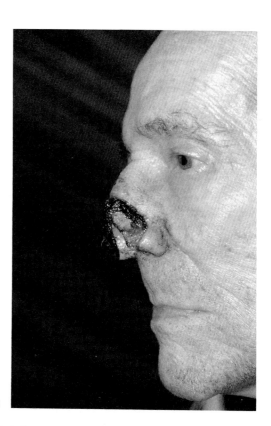

a

b

Figure 1.6. (a, b) Extensive nasal defect on the day of Mohs' surgery with amputation of the entire tip, including cartilages and lining. (c) Basal view after reconstruction of lining and reconstruction of tip projection with multiple conchal cartilage grafts. (d, e) Postoperative views demonstrating good tip projection and contour.

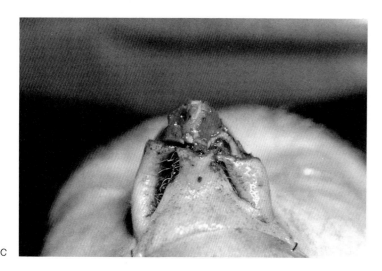

c

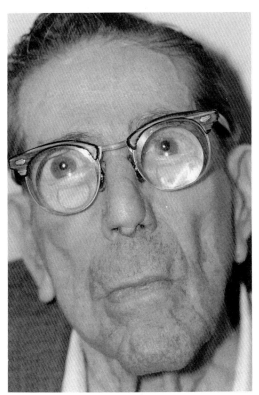

d

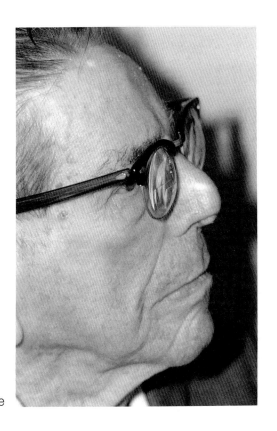

e

Because newly reconstructed nasal tip skin is less pliable than natural, unoperated nasal skin, the reconstructed noses require extraanatomic cartilaginous support for optimal tip projection and for support of key structures such as the alar rims and the internal valve. In general, the aesthetic and functional result of extensive nasal reconstruction will be enhanced by as much rigidity from cartilage grafting as is feasible.[5]

Finally, skin cover is provided by a combination of the pedicled forehead flap with available local flaps. To adapt the forehead flap to wide nasal defects, I prefer to combine the forehead flap with adjacent local flaps to narrow the ultimate nasal defect. In most patients, a 3.5-cm-wide forehead defect can easily be closed; in patients with lax foreheads, this can be widened to 4 cm, but with considerable tension. If the nasal defect is wider than this, I prefer to narrow the nasal defect by recruitment of adjacent cheek flaps rather than to use a larger forehead flap, with an inevitably worse forehead donor site scar. Whenever possible, the forehead flap and combined local flaps should be designed so that each flap reconstructs an entire aesthetic subunit of the nose, and the join lines between the flaps will fall at the margins of the aesthetic subunits.

For very wide nasal defects, I have used cheek advancement flaps, with perialar crescenteric excisions,[5,6] to reconstruct the aesthetic subunits of the nasal sidewalls. Cheek flaps may be elevated in the plane between the subcutaneous fat and the facial muscles and advanced from lateral toward medial to narrow the nasal defect (Figures 1.1b, c, 1.7a, b, 1.8a–d). The superior edge of the cheek flap can be either at the orbital rim (especially in older patients with abnormal snap-back tests or a tendency toward ectropion), or as a subciliary incision (in younger patients with good lower

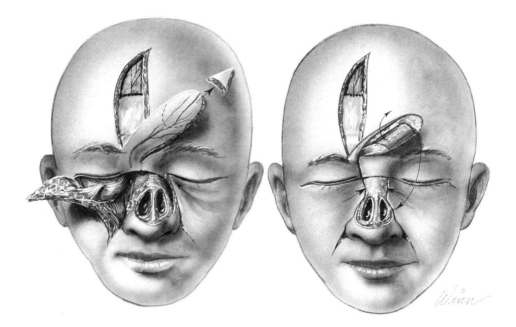

Figure 1.7. (a) Wide nasal defects should be narrowed by lateral to medial cheek advancement flaps. (b) Flaps are undermined in the plane superficial to the facial muscles and advanced from lateral to medial. The superior edge of the flap is either at the orbital rim or at the subciliary line, depending upon the patient's lower lid tone. The inferior margin on the flap extends along the junction of the ala and the cheek and along the nasal-labial crease to the corner of the mouth, then along the "marionnette lines" to the free border of the mandible, if necessary.

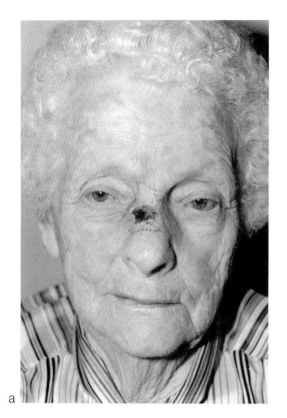

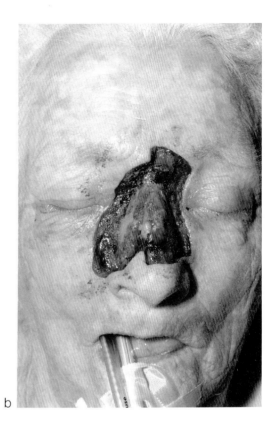

a

b

Figure 1.8. (a) Recurrent ulcerated nasal skin cancer requiring wide excision of almost the entire intercanthal skin. (b) Illustration of post-Mohs' defect down to bare nasal bones, measuring 6.5 cm in width.

(c) Elevation of extensive bilateral cheek flaps for narrowing of the resultant nasal defect. (d) Final result, after secondary division and inset of the forehead flap pedicle.

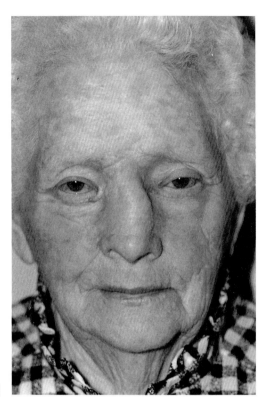

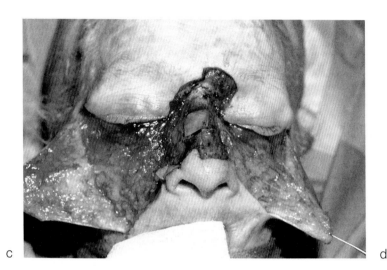

c

d

lid tone). If necessary, the flap may be extended transversely from the lateral orbit to the preauricular crease, and then inferiorly along the preauricular crease to the earlobe, as a total cheek superomedial advancement flap (Figure 1.8a–c). Inferiorly, as the cheek flap advances from lateral to medial it will have excessive vertical height because the cheek is taller laterally than medially. Its excessive height is trimmed as a perialar cresenteric excision along the margin of the remaining nasal alae, and inferolaterally along the nasal-labial crease. The underside of the cheek flap is secured to the nasal bone periosteum or to the upper lateral cartilage to recreate the normal concavity alongside the nose.

When portions of the nasal alae are missing, we reconstruct the nasal ala (and in large defects we discard any small portions of nasal ala that remain) with subcutaneously pedicled, superiorly based nasal-labial flaps. Fortunately, nasal-labial flaps and cheek advancement flaps can both be harvested from the same cheek, using the discarded portion of the cheek, i.e., the perialar crescentic excision, for the alar reconstruction (Figure 1.9a).

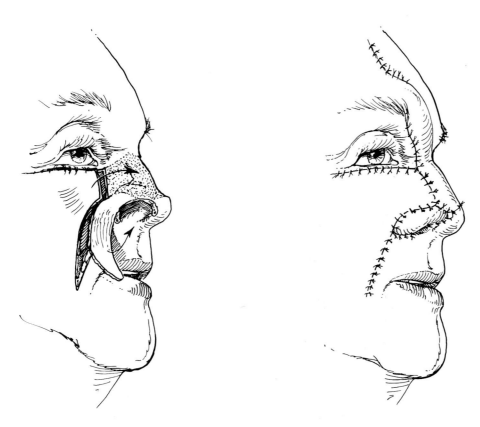

Figure 1.9. (a) Superiorly based, subcutaneous pedicled, nasal-labial flaps may be turned over to provide reconstruction of the entire aesthetic subunit of the missing nasal ala. (b) Anterior columellar defects are reconstructed with a "V-to-Y" advancement of the entire columella with a "Y" closure in the central upper lip.

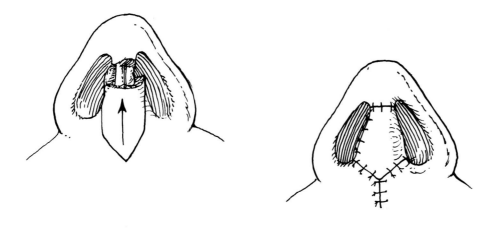

If the anterior portion of the columella also needs reconstruction, the remaining columella is advanced anteriorly as an entire columellar subcutaneous pedicled flap with a "V-Y" closure of the donor site in the upper portion of the upper lip (Figure 1.9b).

Once the existing nasal defect has been narrowed by the advancement of cheek and/or nasal-labial flaps, an exact template is made of the final nasal defect on sterilized, unexposed x-ray film. The template is used to plan the pedicled forehead flap in reverse on the forehead. The point of rotation of the flap is predicted to be the superomedial corner of the orbit. An additional 1 cm of flap length must be allotted to compensate for the loss in length from the 180° twist in the flap from the forehead to the nose. The eventual final skin island within the template must be placed beneath the frontal hairline. In balding patients, this is not a problem; for those with low hairlines and nasal tip defects the forehead flap will reach, but with no extra length. The skin island is centered exactly above the superomedial orbital corner to fall exactly on the course of the supratrochlear neurovascular bundle. The flap base may be severely narrowed at its base, or even designed as an island. The cephalad triangular extension of the flap to allow closure without a dog-ear in the scalp may be run into the hair-bearing scalp as far as necessary to allow for a flat closure.

The forehead flap is designed with the triangular throw-away extension and the cephalad one-half of the flap to be elevated in the subcutaneous plane. At exactly the midpoint of the skin island, the dissection plane is dropped to the subfrontalis or subgaleal plane to 2 cm above the supraorbital rim. At this level the dissection is continued inferiorly in the subperiosteal plane. A wide subperiosteal cuff is incised down to the frontal-nasal suture in the midline and to the orbital roof at approximately the midpoint of the supraorbital rim. This allows a wide cuff of periosteal protection around the origin of the supratrochlear bundle. The periosteum must be cut as a three-sided flap to allow mobilization of this small segment of periosteum downward with the forehead flap.

The secondary forehead defect should be closed prior to insetting the flap onto the nose. The adjacent forehead may be undermined in the subgaleal extraperiosteal plane as far laterally as necessary to allow closure. For extremely wide forehead defects, i.e., those between 3.5 and 4.0 cm in width, immediate intraoperative expansion of the adjacent forehead, using 30-cc balloon Foley catheters, has proved helpful for the extra 0.5-cm deficit in forehead closure. On occasion, galeal scoring is also necessary to allow forehead closure.

Finally, the forehead flap is inset into the residual nasal defect. At least three-quarters of the circumference of the nasal defect can be closed to the forehead flap, leaving open only that portion of the nasal defect directly beneath the center of the flap. The flap is not wide enough to allow it to be tubed on itself. The underside of the flap between its origin and the cephalad margin of the nasal defect is left raw and covered with a dressing only.

The pedicled forehead flap is divided and inset at 3 weeks. A rubber band tourniquet test around the flap can confirm adequate recipient vascularization to the distal end of the flap. At the time of division and inset of the pedicle under local anesthesia, the forehead portion is incised as a minimal inverted "V" to allow repositioning of the medial brow element on the side of the flap. Only the inferior 2 cm of the forehead wound needs to be reopened. At the pedicle inset, the cephalad one-half of the forehead flap should be defatted. This was originally the inferior one-half of the flap, i.e., that portion elevated in the subfrontalis or subgaleal plane. With this defatting at the time of division and inset, the entire flap should have the thickness of forehead skin only and should be comparable in thickness to surrounding nasal skin.

Because of the total division of their vascular and lymphatic supply, the forehead flaps remain slightly edematous for 3 to 6 months after pedicle division. After that time, if the forehead flap is still too thick compared with the contour of the adjacent nasal skin, it can be reelevated and rethinned as appropriate. As much as 50% of the surface of the flap can be elevated and defatted at a single stage.

DISCUSSION

There are multiple advantages in using the pedicled forehead flap for extensive nasal reconstruction, as described above. The major advantage of the forehead flap lies in its color, texture, and thickness as compared with the surrounding nasal skin. Skin grafts and distal flaps will never seem so similar to the residual nasal tissues.

The forehead flap allows the major, if not total, reconstruction of the nose in one stage with immediate reconstruction of lining, structural support, and cover in a single operation, without delay, and immediately following Mohs' excision. Accurate aesthetic reconstruction is much easier at the time of the single-stage reconstruction than in the future when flap edema, scar immobility, and distortion of normal structures all impair accuracy.

The limited-size forehead flap combined with recruitment of adjacent local flaps allows for an improved forehead scar compared with techniques that utilize larger forehead flaps for the entire defect. Forehead defects greater than 4 cm in width are difficult to close primarily. Secondarily healed forehead scars often leave a depression that is difficult to camouflage. Forehead flaps such as the "seagull flap"[7] that provide alar as well as dorsal and sidewall cover also entail significant forehead tightness in closure and difficulties with the resultant scar. The wings of the "seagull" may need a preliminary delay.

The design of the forehead flap, based on a single supratrochlear artery, preserves the opposite supratrochlear neurovascular bundle for use in the future should the need arise for an additional reconstruction.

The opportunity to provide lining reconstruction with adjacent lining tissues, as opposed to turned-in skin, does not compromise the patient's oncologic status by hiding tissues that are subject to future malignant degeneration. This is extremely important for these patients who are prone to recurrent and new primary tumors in any actinically damaged skin.

These complex nasal reconstructions can be performed under local anesthesia, if necessary, without undue difficulty. In this aged population, this is often a marked advantage. The patients' acceptance of local anesthesia is largely determined by their experience with the Mohs' excision under local anesthesia. Those with a good experience were more willing to accept additional surgery under local anesthesia than those who had been frightened or discomforted by their excision.

On the other hand, there are disadvantages to the forehead flap reconstruction. The 3-week interval between initial flap reconstruction and pedicle division is psychologically difficult for most patients. The advance preoperative consultation with the patient has proved extremely useful in emotionally preparing them for the appearance of the flap and for their reaction to it. I would find it very difficult to discuss a reconstruction as complex as a forehead flap with a patient who had already spent the greater portion of the day in the dermatologist's office undergoing Mohs' ablation of much of the nose. The consultation is emotionally traumatic enough when contemplated in advance; on the day of their Mohs' surgery, most patients would be hard-pressed to pay attention to their plastic surgeon's discussion of alternatives.

Because the underside of the flap is left unlined, there is an inevitable ooze that runs down along the patient's face and eyes for 24 to 48 hours postoperatively. For this reason, we have chosen to hospitalize these patients until the bleeding stops spontaneously. This short hospitalization also allows them to emotionally adjust to their appearance and to become comfortable with wound care before going home.

All patients who contemplate this procedure must be warned of the permanent forehead and scalp numbness and paresthesias that result from the sacrifice of the supratrochlear nerve. Patients who require a pedicled buccal mucosal flap for lining reconstruction must also be warned about the resultant oral-nasal fistula. I have offered to close this fistula at the time of pedicle inset in all patients in whom buccal mucosa was used; all have refused, as they find the fistula asymptomatic and undetectable.

CONCLUSION

The axial paramedian forehead flap, based on the supratrochlear neurovascular bundle, provides forehead skin for nasal reconstruction that is a near-perfect match for nasal skin in color, texture, and thickness.

The axial forehead flap nasal reconstruction, extended by the addition of local flaps, cartilage grafts, and lining reconstruction, is adaptable to a wide variety of extensive nasal defects. By reserving the forehead flap for the key central subunits of the nasal dorsum and tip, and by using cheek flaps and nasal-labial flaps for the nasal alae and sidewall reconstructions, even very wide nasal defects may be reconstructed with an acceptable, primarily closed forehead scar. The undelayed axial forehead flap based on the supratrochlear neurovascular bundle is reliable; the vessels are anatomically constant; and the flap provides an excellent match in color, texture, and thickness to the adjacent nasal skin.

ACKNOWLEDGMENT

The author would like to acknowledge his close mutual relationship with Dr. Edward Parry, his colleague in Mohs' dermatology. Without Dr. Parry's cooperation and encouragement, this work would not have been possible.

ROUNDTABLE DISCUSSION

DR. MOSES

In forehead flap nasal reconstruction we must be flexible, because the defects can vary greatly with the variable nature of the tumors and the excisions. The forehead flap should provide the central element of nasal reconstruction, a key aesthetically by providing the central reconstructed element of the nasal dorsum and the tip, as well as a logical "key" as a place to begin. The remaining aesthetic subunits of the nose should be recruited from additional local tissues, if available, such as cheek flaps, nasolabial flaps, and columellar flaps. This enables the forehead defect to be closed primarily with a fine line scar that is barely noticeable in the aged population. Structure needs to be replaced with structure, and lining needs to be replaced with lining.

DR. STAHL

I think that we ought to remember skin grafts in nasal reconstructions. They won't suffice for full-thickness defects, but on many occasions a skin graft from a suitable donor site with suitable thickness can give good results and will also spare flap donor sites for future problems. Secondly, we should consider the option of tissue expansion on the forehead donor site. In cases where you have the luxury of time to accomplish that, expansion can give you more forehead tissue and still allow primary closure of the donor site.

I have also turned down frontalis muscle flaps, draped them over the nose, and put skin grafts on them to give a thin cover with good color match. One other thing that has helped me in the difficult area of columellar reconstruction in cases with contiguous central upper lip defects is extended Abbe flaps with an extension for the columella. However, they require a revision to establish a labiocolumellar angle.

In terms of pitfalls, one precaution in these patients is that they may often get new cutaneous lesions or will have many more, and we have to be careful in selecting our donor sites to prevent transplanting premalignant lesions to reconstructive sites.

DR. ZUBOWICZ

One very useful type of lining that I have used for the lateral nasal vault and the upper lateral cartilages has been a hinged septal mucosal flap, with contralateral mucosa and a plate of septal cartilage brought with it. The cartilage is used to replace the upper lateral cartilage, and the lining from the contralateral side, which is hinged superiorly, replaces the missing lining.

DR. GROTTING

I have been very happy with the addition of the septal pivot flap as described by Burget when trying to reconstruct the cartilaginous vault and to restore adequte tip projection. This has been one of the problems in the past, that is, trying to get a nose where the tip projects above the dorsum. In patients such as you've shown who have had this area completely resected for tumor, the septal pivot flap is an ideal way of adding the amount of additional lining that you need to restore the vestibule of the nose while trying to preserve the function of the nose as well. One of the problems with simply turning down existing mucosa and suturing it is that you have a space between that lining closure and the cartilage framework that you've built on top of it. You've gotten the lining closed, but at the expense of stenosing the vestibule of the nose. The septal pivot flap, when it is available, has solved that problem.

In my experience with younger patients who have thicker skin, reconstructing the nasal sidewall with a cheek advancement flap obliterates the natural angle at the base of the nasal pyramid, and sometimes one loses the important contour there. I have found that putting the scar there and reconstructing both the dorsum and the nasal sidewalls as a continuous subunit has given better aesthetic results.

DR. ELLIOTT

I would like to introduce the subject of introperative expansion of the forehead. I have tried it on a number of occasions and am not impressed by the expansion that is attained. I think that other authors who are even more experienced have demonstrated that intraoperative expansion doesn't recruit much, if any, additional tissue.

Dr. Moses

First, when I advance cheek flaps, I try to advance the cheek flap so that the margin of the cheek flap and the forehead flap lies at the junction of the aesthetic subunits of the nasal dorsum and the nasal sidewalls. This is where the shadowing occurs in an oblique view of the nose. To avoid retraction of the cheek flap and obliteration of the concavity at the cheek–nose junction, I fix the underside of the cheek flap to the periosteum of the nasal bones, or to the upper lateral cartilages, to recreate the sulcus alongside the nose.

Second, regarding expansion, I don't think we get much from intraoperative expansion, but I think that just a little bit can sometimes make a big difference between a wound that is closed and a wound that remains open or dehisces. At most I think I might get a half-centimeter, but sometimes an extra half-centimeter can make a difference.

Dr. MacKinnon

I am not sure I agree about the columellar flaps. I would usually reconstruct the columella with a graft or with an extension of the forehead flap. If you're going to make a forehead incision vertically, anyway, I don't see a reason not to extend the length of the flap to reconstruct the columella too, because it hides it so nicely in shadow under the nose.

Dr. Stahl

The pericranium and/or frontalis flaps can be very helpful to give you a little thin, but significant, margin for protection and allow cover with skin grafts.

Dr. Grotting

What if the forehead is not available and you have the same defect? What do you use?

Dr. Moses

I think that if there was any forehead available I would try to use it. If I couldn't do a pedicled forehead flap, I might try an old-fashioned scalping flap.

DR. ELLIOTT

I think there's another useful variation of the scalping flap: the Washio flap, which takes postauricular skin on the superficial temporal pedicle. It can be made larger, although it is generally described as a fairly small flap. It certainly could be extended down the neck and transferred. Another possiblity is the free flap transfer, but in my experience these are always thick. I don't care which thin flap you use, it is always too thick and bulky. I have not been able to get free flaps to the point where I can legitimately call them thin and nicely aesthetic. Patients tolerate prostheses, but as we all know, if they use them for some time they grow tired of the trouble and are more interested in an autogenous tissue answer.

DR. ZUBOWICZ

I've used the Washio flap on two patients, and I agree that it certainly doesn't give the result that one sometimes sees in drawings. When vascularized tissue is definitely needed and it's not easily sculptable as a forehead flap, I would use it as a last resort.

DR. ELLIOTT

When the hinged septal flaps are used, how often do nasal septal perforations necessitate treatment?

DR. MOSES

One hundred percent of the patients have nasal septal perforations. It is inherent in the design of the flap, but in my experience, none of them have been symptomatic, so none have requested or required treatment. The beauty of the hinge flap is that the cartilage that comes with the flap is actually vascularized cartilage.

DR. ELLIOTT

What about some of the flaps from antiquity, like Tagliacozzi's upper arm flap? Do you ever use that?

DR. MOSES

No, but I think it was a great flap in the fifteenth century.

Dr. Stahl

I am curious why you wait so long before dividing the pedicle of the forehead flap? It has been my experience that much less than 3 weeks was adequate.

Dr. Moses

If I have any doubt about the revascularization of the flap from its distal end, I do a rubber-band tourniquet test to see if the flap has revascularized its distal end before I divide it. Three weeks has always been sufficient time; several patients needed the full 3 weeks to have a positive tourniquet test. I don't feel any great rush to do it any sooner.

Dr. Zubowicz

I think that 3 weeks is too conservative. I think you can divide them in 7 to 10 days, and I think that's even a bit conservative.

Dr. Moses

Most of these flaps have cartilage grafts in between the flap and the recipient bed, so that they may not be getting surface-to-surface revascularization but just neovascularization from the periphery.

Dr. Elliott

If this is an axial flap, why can't you make it an island flap and not worry about the pedicle division?

Dr. Moses

You can make it an island flap, and in 3 of the 16 cases I did, it was an island flap. The subcutaneous pedicle was so thick that then I wanted to go back and divide it anyway.

Dr. Grotting

I think that's an important point. The second operation is more than just dividing the pedicle, it's contouring and insetting. I think the important part of the division and inset is elevating the flap and defatting it as much as possible to get very thin coverage over your cartilage framework.

Dr. Moses

Do you actually elevate all of the flap?

Dr. Grotting

No, obviously you can't elevate all of the flap and cut the pedicle at the same time, but you can elevate very near to the distal marginal inset and defat 85% of it and it will live.

References

1. Soutar OS, Elliot D, Rao GSS. Buccal mucosal flaps in nasal reconstruction. Br J Plast Surg 1990; 43:612–616.

2. Burget GC, Menick FJ. Nasal support and lining: The marriage of beauty and blood supply. Plast Reconstr Surg 1989;84:189–203.

3. Burget GC, Menick FJ. Nasal reconstruction: Seeking a fourth dimension. Plast Reconstr Surg 1986;78:145–157.

4. Menick FJ. Aesthetic refinements in use of forehead for nasal reconstruction: The paramedian forehead flap. Clin Plast Surg 1990;17:607–622.

5. Burget GC, Menick FJ. Aesthetic Reconstruction of the Nose. St. Louis: Mosby–Year Book Inc., 1994.

6. Webster JP. Crescentic peri-alar cheek excision for upper lip flap advancement with a short history of upper lip repair. Plast Reconstr Surg 1955;16:434–464.

7. Millard DR Jr. Reconstructive rhinoplasty for the lower half of a nose. Plast Reconstr Surg 1974;53:133–139.

ABBE FLAP FOR LIP RECONSTRUCTION

McKay McKinnon

THE PROBLEM

The patient presented with a long-standing philtral deformity character-ized by (1) a deep Tennison-type scar crossing the center of the philtrum, (2) a retrusive upper lip, (3) mild transverse tightness, and (4) single arc of vermilion, lacking any cupid's bow (the "chapeau de gendarme" lip). Also complicating the lip abnormalities were an angle class III malocclusion, maxillary insufficiency, missing central and lateral incisors, nasal septal deviation, an oronasal fistula, a vertically short lower lip, an acute labio-mental crease, and pseudoprognathism.

INTRODUCTION

The long and colorful history of the Abbe-Stein-Sabattini flap has seen several refinements. There remains, though, a sizable segment of surgeons who are still reluctant to use this flap when faced with severe upper lip and philtral deformities. In the repaired bilateral or unilateral cleft lip with transverse tightness, vertical shortness, or contour irregularity of the philtrum and vermilion, one should consider the Abbe flap as the bull's-eye shot toward an elusive target—the ideal normal philtrum .

The surgical strategy of the illustrated case included three stages:

1. 7-mm maxillary advancement, malar bone graft augmentation, alveoloplasty (with bone graft) and fistula closure;
2. Abbe flap with division and inset 10 days later;
3. rhinoplasty, genioplasty (reduction), revision of Abbe flap vermilion, and dermabrasion of scars.

Anatomy

The precise contour and anatomy of the ideal normal upper lip with its proportions and position relative to the rest of the mouth and face should be understood. The dimensions of the normal infant, child, and adult philtrum should be a standard reference point. Sex and race should also be considered.

The Abbe flap is a composite flap of skin, muscle, mucosa, and vermilion. Although it could probably include bone and even teeth, this appears unnecessary in practice. Millard has built a powerful case that Abbe flaps should be precisely midline in their origin and insertion. The only exception to that rule occurs when the upper lip defect is lateral to the philtral column and, even here, the Abbe is often preferable to an Estlander flap.

The Abbe flap has sometimes been successful as a composite graft, but the putative advantages of this are outweighed, I think, by the risks of only having a ``one-shot'' attempt at hitting the surgical target. The position of the coronal branch of the labial artery, which is highly consistent, should be known and sought out almost down to the vessel itself. For this flap thinness of the pedicle is useful and desirable.

Technique

A precise, midline, upper lip incision is marked from the base of the columella to the vermilion border (Figure 2.1). The existing scar is ignored in

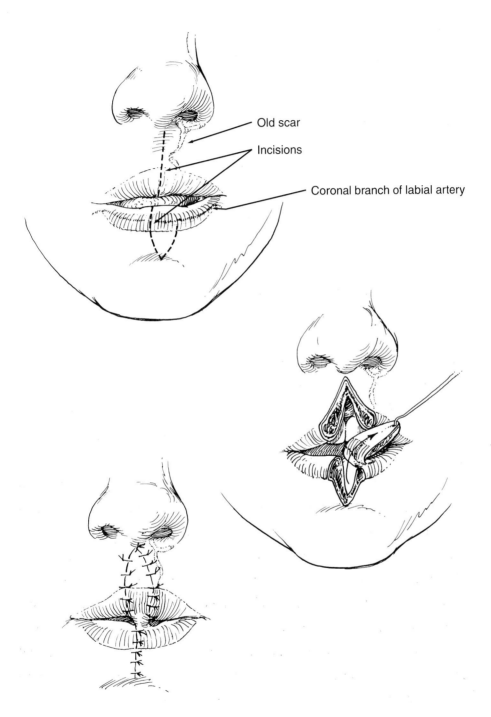

Figure 2.1. Technique for transposition of Abbe flap.

the patient with unilateral cleft lip. The upper lip vermilion is slightly fuller on the patient's left side, and this will eventually need to be adjusted. The height of the flap will be 18 mm measured from the columellar base to the mucocutaneous junction. The ideal philtral width for this patient was judged to be 12 mm. The Abbe flap is drawn in the shape of a shield along the skin and mucosa. Because the lower lip's natural pout will not be automatically transferred with the Abbe flap, adequate mucosal height is important to allow relaxation for an eventual upper lip pout by secondary revision. The amount of upper incisor shown (ideally, 1 to 3 mm) should be determined from the current lip height, the already repositioned maxilla, the presence of dental hardware, the need for later dental bonding, capping, or prosthetics, and the desired Abbe flap height.

The Abbe flap incisions are made by first scoring the skin and vermilion, followed with a No. 11 blade as a full-thickness incision while the assistant reveals the extended lip and mucosa held by skin hooks. The position of the divided labial artery is noted. With a No. 15 blade and/or Joseph scissors, a narrowing of the pedicle follows with an incision freeing the mucocutaneous junction on the side of the pedicle. A 3- to 5-mm diameter pedicle will allow greatest ease of transposition with less risk of flap congestion following the 180° turn. The mucosal 5-0 chromic sutures are first placed, then the muscle is repaired. If the recipient area is heavily scarred, some freeing of the orbicularis may be necessary. The apical skin stitch should be a perfect join to the columella base. Since the upper lip is triangulated and the Abbe flap is cut in a shield shape, the final three-dimensional shape will require some trimming at the columellar junction to maintain a natural curve of the philtral column. If the patient with unilateral cleft lip has a strong normal side philtrum leading into the medial one-third of the nostril sill instead of toward the columella, the apex of the Abbe flap can be blunted to "straighten" the upper portion of the columns. I find this preferable to the more artificial appearance of the "W" or split-tail Abbe flap.

The color of the flap is usually bluish when the final insetting sutures are placed. Nevertheless, the blanch test should still show prompt color return. White flaps demand suture removal, pedicle alteration, or both.

With general anesthesia, nasogastric suctioning lessens the risk of postoperative emesis, and I hold the jaw during emergence from anesthesia. An awake patient, either a child or an adult, will be less likely to injure the flap inadvertently. I do not use bandages, splints, or intermaxillary fixation.

CASE 1 (FIGURE 2.2)

This patient had routine flap division as an office procedure 10 days postoperatively. A final trimming and revision of the vermilion borders was performed 2 months later at the time of rhinoplasty and reduction genioplasty. She also developed an area of hypertrophic scarring near the flap apex. This was initially a little worrisome, but with time and a small dermabrasion at the time of genioplasty, it proved to be inconspicuous. The patient developed full motion and sensation to the Abbe flap in approximately 4 months.

The original cleft scar diminished with relaxation of the lip. The successful illusion of the Abbe flap is that it is the rightful occupant of the philtrum. The addition of pout, movement, and a nearly normal relationship to the rest of the upper and lower lips further diminishes the presence of three new scars. A lateral view reveals that the upper lip has finally emerged in front of the cheek. Even with the 7-mm Le Fort I could not achieve this relationship.

DISCUSSION

The patient with secondary unilateral cleft lip represents a problem that makes many surgeons continue to fear using the Abbe flap. This fear stems from the uncertainty of new scars and the problem of symmetry. But although the patient may understandably balk at the idea of a new scar on the lower lip, the surgeon should realize that the new scar is warranted to restore a deformed lip to near normal form and shape. The Abbe flap is

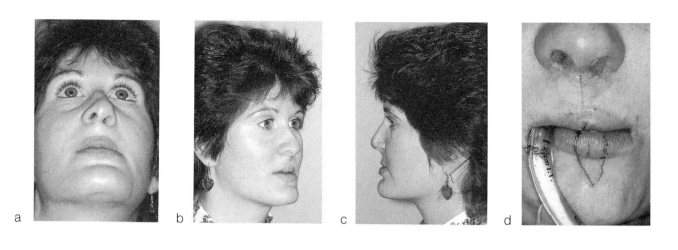

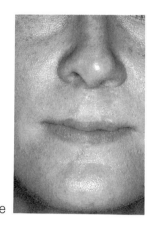

Figure 2.2.(a-i)(Case 1). Patient with left complete unilateral cleft lip following a triangular repair, now with wide scar and deficient philtrum. She underwent Le Fort I advancement and genioplasty and subsequent Abbe flap.

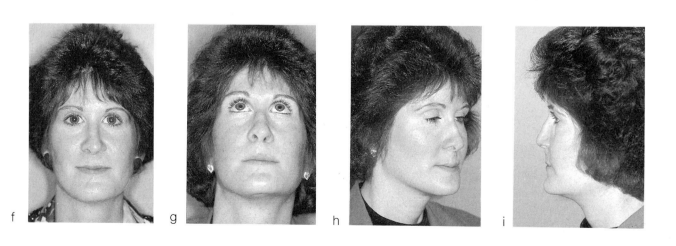

well-suited for the reconstruction of normal philtral height and width, lip contour, and dynamism. If these goals can be achieved, the concern for new scars will become a deservedly secondary consideration. Smaller flaps or grafts cannot compete with the quality of Abbe flaps where composite deficiencies are present.

The case presented of the unilateral cleft lip invites further scrutiny of the use of the Abbe flap because of the resulting hypertrophic scarring over part of it. The point to reemphasize is that the new scarring should not deter resort to the Abbe flap when new contour, near normal landmarks, and a tension-free pout can be obtained. The answer to the question of what to do with the original scar varies from nothing to complete incorporation into the Abbe flap—so long as the Abbe flap retains its ideal dimensions and central position. For the bilateral cleft lip requiring an Abbe flap reconstruction, the flap width should still not exceed the normal lip philtrum dimensions. If transverse lip tension persists, consider perialar relaxing incisions over widening the Abbe flap or, worse, leaving the existing two scars and insetting the Abbe flap with two new scars.

CASE 2 (FIGURE 2.3)

Nonstandard shapes and composites of the Abbe flap can be used for individual patients. The case shown reveals an Abbe flap with philtral columns that are directed more toward the nostril sill than the columella. For patients who have good skin scars but poor vermilion and/or orbicularis, the Abbe flap with the muscle and vermilion only may be preferable. If the entire upper lip vermilion is deficient, then the "fleur de lis" Abbe, as first described by Millard, can be used.

In conclusion, the Abbe flap is a "one-shot" effort and the surgeon must be able to resort to it with confidence in its viability. Any flap can be mortally injured, but the Abbe flap is more resilient than most axial flaps by virtue of its predictable, healthy blood supply, relatively short dimensions, and transposition to a well-vascularized bed. Even preexistent lip pits will not deter its successful use.

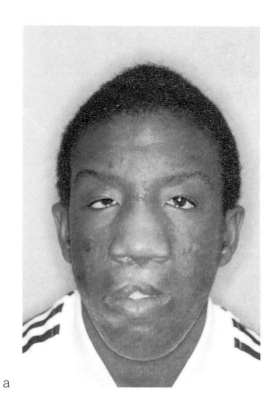

a

Figure 2.3.(a-d)(Case 2). Bilateral cleft lip deformity with maxillary insufficiency, mandibular prognathism, and macroretrogenia. Three-year result after Le Fort I advancement, sagittal split mandibulotomy, genioplasty, and Abbe flap at one operation. Patient had subsequent blepharoptosis correction.

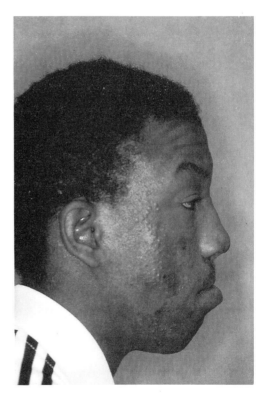

b

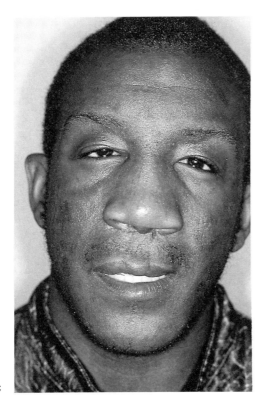

c

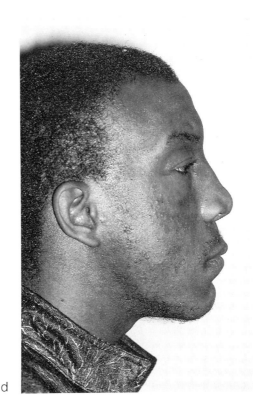

d

ROUNDTABLE DISCUSSION

DR. McKINNON

The discussion of this case still goes back to the controversy over using an Abbe flap for unilateral cleft lip. It is a very hard decision for the surgeon who created the original lip repair to make because it admits to failure of the original technique as a solution to the problem. The Abbe flap has overwhelming advantages over other flaps that are of lesser risk and lesser extent, because of these three reasons:

1. It provides new landmarks that are within the control of the surgeon.
2. It provides anterior projection and compound tissue, which are usually missing to some degree in patients with cleft lip.
3. It provides dynamic action.

DR. STAHL

I want to raise the issue of the design of the flap. Whether it's for a cleft or tumor defect, there is a tendency to make the flap wider than the normal central lip segment is, and I think that we should strive to make these fairly narrow. There are some guidelines as to how wide the normal distance is between philtral columns. Based on the data from *Cleft Craft*, Volume II, (p. 36) the distance is 7 to 13 mm in adult women and 10 to 16 mm in adult men.

DR. ZUBOWICZ

Some patients with unilateral cleft lip certainly don't need anything. It may be difficult, outside of a small scar, to tell whether or not they had ever had a problem. Other patients, both with bilateral clefts and some with unilateral clefts, have marked restriction in vertical height and look tight. In some cases the selection of Abbe flaps, such as in this case, is pretty easy to make, but what about the gray area? Do you have any suggestions as to when an Abbe flap is too much to use?

DR. McKINNON

I agree with Dr. Stahl that the majority of Abbe flaps are too wide, and the majority of cleft lip repairs are too wide. The most common Abbe flaps are used for bilateral cleft lip, of course, and the usual goal is to replace the original prolabial tissue. Too little consideration is given, though, to providing ideal philatral dimensions. For these reasons, I prefer to make primary bilateral cleft lip repairs as narrow as possible. Also, the secondary Abbe flap repair for unilateral clefts should err on the side of minimal width as well, ignoring the possibility of excising the scar of the original repair. The temptation to extend the Abbe flap so as to excise the original scar should probably be resisted, as Millard has suggested.

Dr. Zubowicz, there are many indications for the Abbe flap, but you are asking where the borderline is. I think it has to be a problem with composite deficiencies. There is rarely a case that has landmarks only that are so badly distorted that it demands an Abbe flap. The same is true for lip retrusion—it rarely stands alone as a justification for the Abbe flap. Lesser procedures with small flaps or grafts, or even alveolar cleft bone grafting, can improve the retrusion alone. The issue of dynamism in a cleft lip is a hard one to judge, because few patients realize how dynamic or adynamic their lips are. I think when all three of these areas, i.e., landmarks, projection, and dynamism, come into play, it becomes a less gray issue. Furthermore, if the philtral dimensions are good but there is poor projection and motion, I may do a mucosa-and-muscle-only Abbe flap.

Dr. Toth

Dr. McKinnon, no one can argue with the quality of your results in these two cases, because they are truly excellent.

There are two issues that I want to raise: (1) the issue of the ideal age at which one should consider an Abbe flap, and (2) your timing of Le Forte I advancement prior to releasing the soft tissue and providing augmentation of the upper lip. In the moderate type of deformity in your first patient and in the older patient, I find it very difficult to subject them to the additional scarring that an Abbe flap would provide. The additional scarring of the donor defect, as well as the bilateral upper lip scar are difficult in a 16- or 17-year-old patient. They are very concerned about their appearance in front of other people, and we know full well that it will take at least a year for the scars to settle down. It is a very difficult time of their lives to subject them to bilateral upper lip scarring. Second, it would be my inclination to deal with the soft tissue deformity in the post cleft lip syndrome first, in order to avoid some of the soft tissue forces that can cause relapse in the Le Fort I advancement.

DR. MCKINNON

Those are good points, and I think that it is hard to know what is the best age for doing an Abbe flap. It needs to be a case-by-case judgment. Although I know of reports of Abbe flaps done in the first year of life, that seems to me to make little sense with so many changes yet to come. Even stretching a very small philtrum is still probably a better solution than doing a primary Abbe flap, and I think most surgeons would agree on that.

The question of timing primarily affects teenagers, who present most frequently with the need for an Abbe flap, or something else drastically different for their philtrum. You're right: they've been through multiple operations, maybe 10 years of orthodontia; they've concentrated for lengthy stretches just on the scar itself; and here you're offering them three new ones and not taking away the old one. It can be a very traumatic decision for them and their families. The best approach is to be convinced in your own mind of the potential for an Abbe flap when you have an obviously deformed philtrum that cannot be radically altered in any other way. I deemphasize the new scars, troublesome as they may be for a few months, and emphasize the permanent improvement in lip contour, projection and dynamism. As far as timing of the Le Fort I with the Abbe flap is concerned, I think that that is a judgment call. When I see a lip that is obviously tight, I consider that the Abbe flap may facilitate the Le Fort I advancement, and I may do it even at the same time as the Le Fort I. Although that may seem to be a high-wire act, I have done it on three occasions without complications.

DR. GROTTING

One criticism of the single Abbe flap is that it rotates up. You can get asymmetry between the two sides of the scar. It has been suggested that you can handle this by doing two smaller Abbe flaps rotated toward each other. The obvious disadvantage of this is a midline scar, but sometimes that midline scar can give a better simulation of a philtral dimple than the occasional chronic edema in a single Abbe flap. I have no personal experience with that.

The congested Abbe flap, of course, is a great concern. You have this precious piece of tissue that you want to survive if at all possible and they will, in fact, survive even if you damage the axial artery. Almost always the problem is venous congestion, and I have cooled these flaps postoperatively for the first 48 hours. I think that some of the revascularization occurs very rapidly in this area and perhaps it takes partially as a composite graft. Nitro-paste is also a possibility for the congested Abbe flap.

DR. TOTH

Dr. Grotting mentions the possibility of a composite graft rather than this being a composite flap. We know from other experiences that we can gener-ally take a 1 × 1 cm graft of nearly anything, without providing a blood sup-ply, if we are putting it in a good recipient site and that it will likely survive. I wonder in many instances, as we are skeletonizing the pedicle, whether we are creating a bigger problem by having no venous drainage and an artery pumping into this flap. Perhaps we would be better off just taking it as a free composite graft and avoiding the secondary division procedure?

My other concern is that I need one, or sometimes two, secondary proce-dures to get the Abbe flap right. I generally have too much projection of the central upper lip and I need additional refinement with the excess vermilion. It is important for the patient to know that the potential for one or two sec-ondary procedures is part and parcel of the reconstructive procedure.

DR. MOSES

I have a couple of observations: (1) We have all agreed that the Abbe flap is more typically used for the late bilateral cleft lip deformity than for the late unilateral cleft deformity. I think that this is because most modern repairs of unilateral cleft lips utilize a repair that accurately relocates the normal upper lip philtral dimple, so the Abbe flap is indicated for tightness but not for ab-sence of the philtral dimple. On the other hand, the triangular flap repair that this patient originally had is a repair that does not accurately relocate the philtral dimple, so not so much is lost by throwing away the central seg-ment of the upper lip after this repair as, for example, after a Millard lip re-pair. Regarding planning issues, I would think that tightness of the upper lip is a double-edged sword. The most common indication for the Abbe flap is a tight upper lip, but we have all said that Abbe flaps that are too wide look abnormal. Yet if you do an Abbe flap that is too narrow, you have often not relieved the tightness adequately, so there is a little bit of "damned if you do, damned if you don't." The wider the flap, the better the improvement of the tightness, but the more abnormal the flap might look. It is ultimately the sur-geon's aesthetic judgment.

I also have some difference of opinion regarding the anesthetic management of patients with Abbe flaps. I think that Abbe flaps performed under general anesthesia have a significant risk of avulsion of the flap at the time of awakening from the anesthesia. In children this is not an issue because local anesthesia is not possible. But for adults with Abbe flaps, I think local anesthesia with sedation is much preferable to avoid that uncontrolled period of awakening from general anesthesia where the patient might awake, open his or her mouth, and undo the entire operation. For this same reason, I would refuse to combine an Abbe flap with a complicated intraoral procedure that might be subject to postoperative bleeding, secretions, or swelling in a mouth that will limit access. Having general anesthesia and bleeding in a mouth that can't open is a bad combination.

Finally, one technical point: the lower lip scar is best if it doesn't cross the transverse crease between the lower lip and the chin. For this, sometimes it is best done with a "W" at the bottom rather than as a pennant flap closing to a line that extends below the lower lip crease.

Dr. Stahl

I share the opinion that local anesthesia with good sedation is preferable. I have had pretty good luck with talking to my patients preoperatively about what to expect when they wake up and what they should and should not do. I find that if I mention it to them a couple of times before the preoperative visit, and then right before induction of anesthesia, the prehypnotic suggestion helps the cooperative patient remain cooperative, even during reversal of the anesthesia.

One issue that I do not recall our addressing is the timing of the flap's pedicle division. I think, that this flap could virtually be done as a composite graft and it is not necessary for us to keep the patient's pedicle attached for an excessively long time. Consequently, I think it is safe to divide the pedicle fairly early, such as in 5 days to a week, and not necessarily wait 9 or 10 days.

Dr. Grotting

I think it is probably safe to divide it in 5 days, but I'm not sure whether I would do much insetting or revision at that time. However, it's the tethering of the two lips together that bothers the patient. Perhaps one should simply cut the pedicle at that time and then leave it until we've had more healing before we do any final insetting.

Dr. McKinnon

There are many technical issues, some of which have been raised in the text and some of which have been reemphasized in the discussion. This is a technically demanding operation, and it is obviously in a conspicuous area. The one general question we ought to address, which Dr. Zubowicz raised, is what other tissue could work as well. The only other tissue that I know that would work as well is someone else's upper lip, but we haven't yet gotten to the point of making that possible. I don't think that distant tissue could possibly match the composite characteristics of the Abbe flap. Perhaps soft tissue expansion also deserves more investigation.

The use of an Abbe flap as a graft is well studied and the disadvantages have been described by Millard. I think that if a patient has been waiting 20 years to have this major reconstruction, he or she can be encouraged without much trouble to put up with 10 days of having his or her lips sewn together. I am still traditional about that. Dr. Grotting brought up the question of vessel damage and how the "take" can be enhanced. I am not sure that even those who are skilled in microvascular techniques could salvage a single vessel of such a narrow pedicle if it were damaged. I would probably resort to a free graft if I thought that the vessel was terribly damaged or return it to its original position and go to "plan B." The possibility of using two flaps is an old one, and the results, at least in the older literature, would suggest that the price one pays for a vertical midline scar is not worth the risk. Two Abbe flaps are still not better than one.

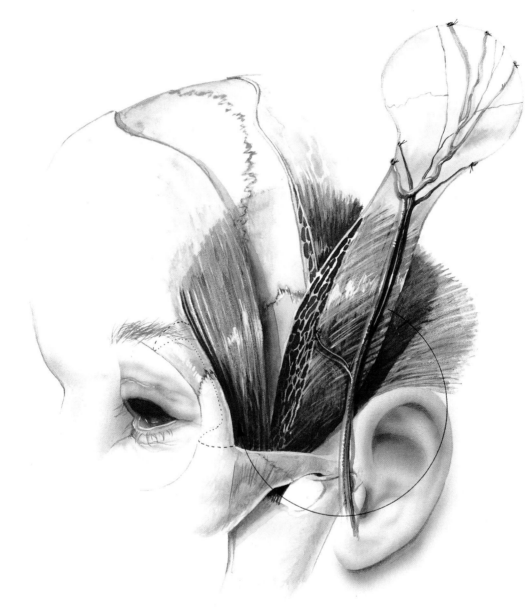

3

Head and Neck Reconstruction with the Temporal Muscle

McKay McKinnon

The Problem

This 7-year-old girl presented with a left orbital rhabdomyosarcoma that persisted despite chemotherapy and radiotherapy (Figure 3.1a). There was no evidence of bone involvement by computed tomographic (CT) scan, and the tumor appeared to be confined to the intraconal tissues. There was moderate proptosis of the globe and considerable ptosis of the upper lid.

Introduction

The temporal muscle is an underused resource for a myriad of head and neck reconstructive problems (Figure 3.2). It offers a wide array of reconstructive possibilities because of its size, unique shape, blood supply, and its ability to rotate in an arc of 360°. Its usefulness is expanded by the possibility of combining it with underlying bone or overlying aponeurosis, fascia, fat, or scalp. For problems involving a deficiency of bone, ear perichondrium, periorbitum, dura mater, facial muscle, fat, subcutaneous tissue, or skin, the temporal muscle continues to be a primary option.

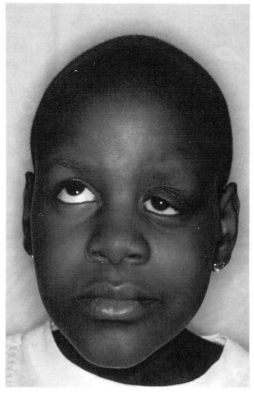

a

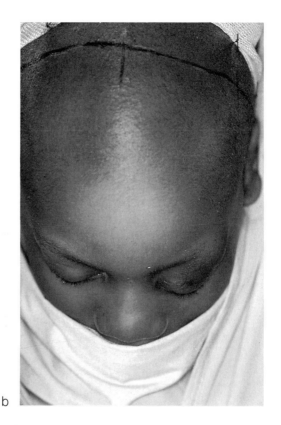

b

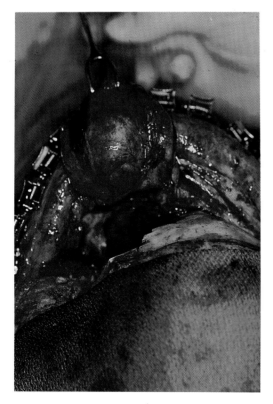

c

Figure 3.1.(a-g). Resection of orbital rhabdomyosarcoma via coronal approach, large orbitotomy, transposition of pericranial/temporalis flap, immediate skin grafting over temporary prosthesis, and 5-year result.

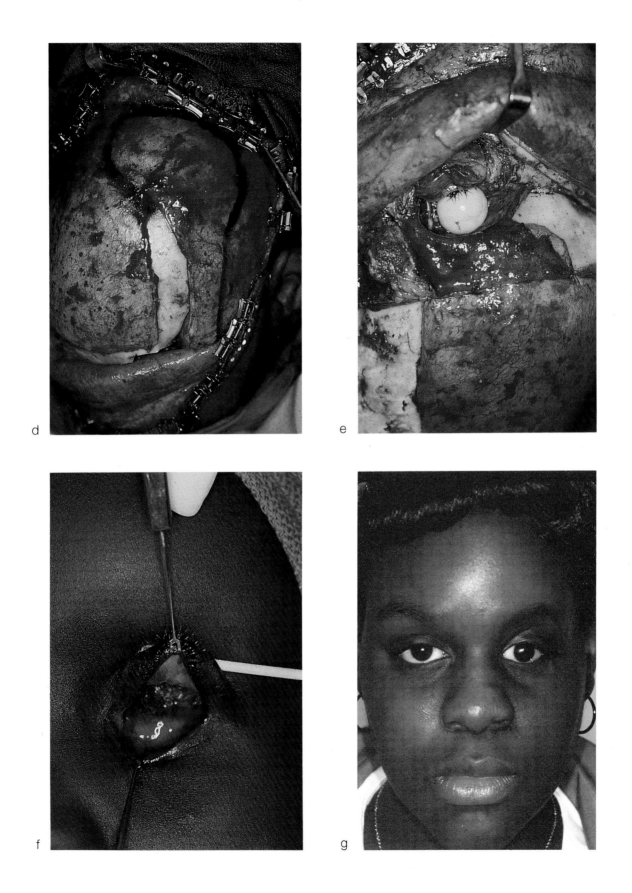

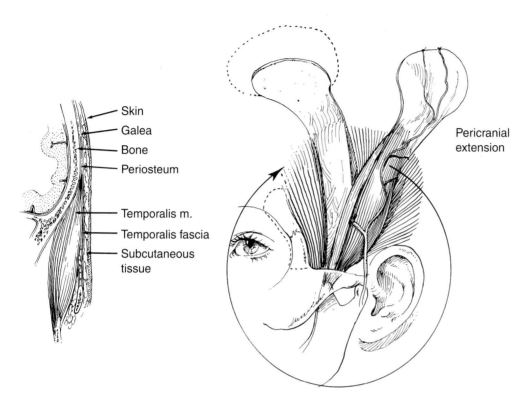

Figure 3.2. Temporal flap vascularized by deep and/or superficial temporal arteries.

ANATOMY

The temporal muscle is two-thirds covered by hair-bearing scalp, is flat posteriorly and thick anteriorly, and ranges in length from origin to insertion (from 10 to 16 cm in the adult). The anterior surface consists of a thin, well-vascularized temporal fascia with a thick underlying aponeurosis[1] over the muscle itself. The aponeurosis is a double layer and between its two layers is the 2- to 3-cm-diameter adipocellular tissue, the "cis sarcosis" of Bichat.[2] The vascular pedicle is tripartite. The superficial temporal artery arises predictably just above the posterior one-third of the zygomatic arch, and two deep pedicles from the internal maxillary artery enter from below. All of these vessels are longitudinally oriented, as are the nerves to the muscle emanating from the mandibular nerve, situated deep to the muscle at its base. The temporal and parietal bones underlying the temporal muscle are mainly supplied by the middle meningeal artery, but the bone has clinically been shown to be capable of vascular transposition via a retained attachment to its overlying temporal muscle.[3]

The temporal muscle, or any part of it, is capable of transposition through a 360° arc. Detachment of the muscle from the coronoid process of the mandible is not usually necessary for flap transposition. The zygomatic arch may be removed to allow an inferior transposition of the muscle and then should be returned to its original position. Great care should be taken in this dissection to avoid injury to the frontal branch of the VIIth nerve, which just overlies and crosses the zygomatic arch and temporal fascia. Beneath the zygomatic arch, the masseter muscle is the major obstacle to transposition. The temporal muscle can reach the medial wall of the ipsilateral orbit as well as the palatal or mandibular midlines, giving an effective length of transfer of approximately 15 cm. For most reconstructive needs, it is usually unnecessary to transpose the entire muscle. The remaining muscle may then be used to recontour the visible temporal hollow and avoid any unsightly depression.

The coronal incision (sometimes referred to as bicoronal) is the safest and easiest approach to the temporal muscle and its components. The standard neurosurgical incision to approach the temporal bone is, unfortunately, an approach that may easily compromise the future use of the muscle for reconstructive purposes, and that does not allow access to the full dimensions of the muscle for one-stage reconstructive procedures.

TECHNIQUE (FIGURE 3.1b-g)

In this case, the surgical goal was to remove the rhabdomyosarcoma and, if possible, preserve lid structures. The surgical strategy was to approach the left orbit through a coronal incision. The patient had postchemotherapy alopecia. The dissection (Figure 3.3) in a subgaleal plane preserved the temporal fascia as well as the underlying aponeurosis and temporal muscle. At the level of the mid-brow, the dissection was carried subpe-

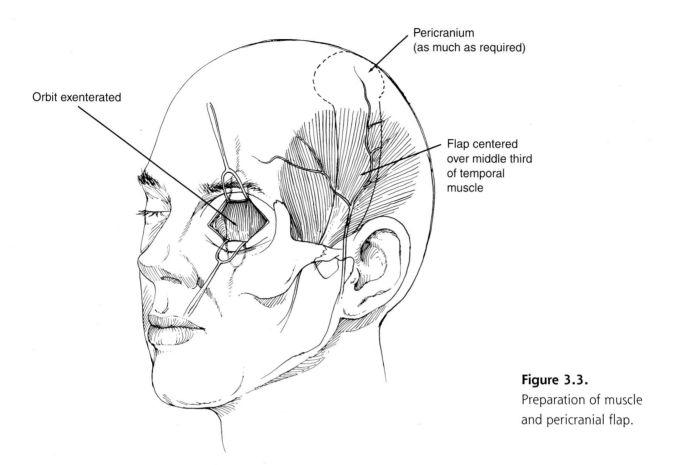

Orbit exenterated

Pericranium
(as much as required)

Flap centered
over middle third
of temporal
muscle

Figure 3.3.
Preparation of muscle
and pericranial flap.

riosteally to the orbit. A large superolateral orbitomy was used for exenteration of the orbital contents, including the bulbar conjunctiva up to the fornices of the upper and lower lids with a sparing of the remainder of the lids. With the assistance of Dr. Marilyn Mets, an ophthalmologist, the removal of the globe and the intraconal contents was completed. The tumor mass was adjacent to the globe and was attached to, but did not extend through, the periosteum. The bony orbit was completely stripped of its periosteum. Biopsies of remaining soft tissue closest to the specimen proved to be free of tumor.

The reconstructive strategy at this point was to lift the orbit with thin vascularized tissue which would permit the immediate placement of a permanent ball prosthesis. The temporal muscle itself is easily long enough to suffice for this purpose and was completely preserved in the field. The attached pericranium just distal to the temporal muscle and vascularized with the muscle itself could provide an even thinner tissue with which to line the orbital cavity. Therefore, a flap was outlined along the left parietal pericranium (Figure 3.3) and the attached temporal muscle using only one-third of the muscle width. The access to the orbital cavity was already provided by the large orbitotomy of the superolateral wall, but the final access would become a window created in this orbitotomy segment so that the muscle and pericranium could be delivered easily behind the lateral orbital rim (Figure 3.4).

The length of temporal muscle is divided longitudinally down to the zygomatic arch. Because the temporal muscle is much broader at its superior origin on the parietal bone than its relatively narrow (but thicker) base in the region near the zygomatic arch, care must be taken to maintain a line of division of the flap so as to preserve the longitudinally oriented vessels within it. Digital manipulation of the flap lessens the chance of injury to the vessels in the flap. The flap is delivered into the orbital cavity with vir-

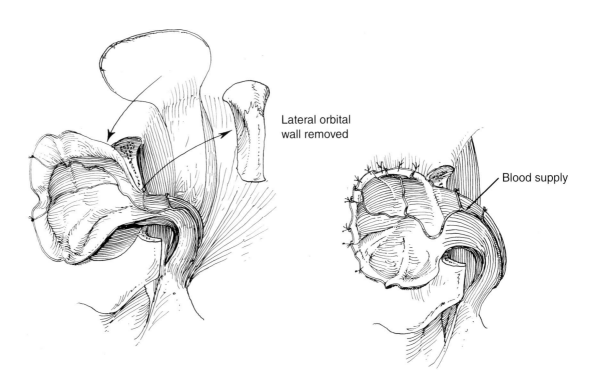

Figure 3.4. Orbital transposition of pericranial temporal muscle flap.

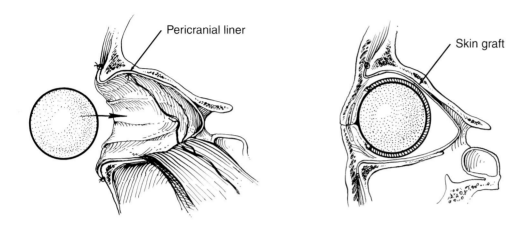

Figure 3.5. Immediate insertion of prosthesis wrapped by skin graft.

tually any-sized pericranial paddle desired, as long as there is an adequate window through the lateral orbital wall. The pericranium in this case was draped in a spherical manner to reconstruct the missing periorbitum with overlap of the orbital rim and frontal bone. A few tacking sutures of Vicryl are helpful to maintain its position. The completion of the reconstruction required the application of a thin, split-thickness skin graft that encircled the spherical implant (Figure 3.5) and was sutured to the palpebral conjunctiva and the pericranium. The orbitotomy was resecured into position with interosseous wires. The posterior two-thirds of the remaining temporal muscle and its overlying aponeurosis were transposed anteriorly to make up for any loss of contour of the temporal hollow in front of the hairline. An attempt should be made to resecure the muscle to the temporal crest (with drill holes placed through the bone of the crest), to a preserved strip of pericranium, or to both. In this way, the final donor site for the temporal muscle is limited to an area beneath hair-bearing scalp and is posteriorly positioned so that no contour deformity can be detected.

Discussion

Other options in this case include the galea frontalis flap, based on supraorbital and supratrochlear vessels. There is a more generous blood supply in virtually every case to flaps based on the temporal muscle than to galea frontalis flaps. In this case, since there was prior radiation therapy of greater than 5000 rad, the possible injury to the frontal, orbital, and supratrochlear vessels could have compromised the galea frontalis flap. Deformity of the brow contour and mobility further mitigate against this flap as a primary choice. In addition, the possibility exists for future readvancement of the temporal muscle into the orbit or any part of it through the same coronal approach. Should the need for bone grafting arise, as it did in this case approximately 6 months after the primary procedure, the temporal muscle again could serve as thick cover for the reconstruction required of the orbital roof and rim.

Objections have been made in the ophthalmologic literature to using temporal muscle flaps to reconstruct the orbit. These objections stem from the possible hindrance to detection of recurrence of tumor, which could be life-threatening. Because this composite pericranial/muscle flap allows the transposition of the very thin, yet highly vascular layer of pericranium immediately adjacent to the temporal muscle origin, there is less likelihood that a tumor recurrence would go undetected in the orbit. Interval CT scan follow-up with 1.5-mm cuts should detect recurrence without regard to the reconstructive method chosen.

Temporal muscle without pericranium has often been used to "fill up" the exenterated orbit, but the thickness of this or any muscle does not allow for further reconstruction with an ocular prosthesis.[4] In those cases, a black patch is usually the final solution.

A third option in this case might have been temporal fascia and/or aponeurosis. The blood supply to the superficial fascia is from the superficial temporal artery. Flap length is less than 15 cm. The temporal muscle can vascularize underlying cranial bone, which can provide a composite flap to the orbit. This concept has particular application where (1) bone is absent or removed as specimen, (2) radiation therapy will follow surgery, and (3) a thicker reconstruction between brain and orbit is desirable.

ROUNDTABLE DISCUSSION

DR. MOSES

In this case, you used the pericranium extension based on the vascular pedicle of the temporalis muscle. One of the disadvantages of using the muscle as the vascular pedicle for the ultimate piece of pericranium is the temporal hollow that results. What advantage did you get with the use of this technique as compared to a pedicle of the temporoparietal fascia in which there would not have been sacrifice of the function of the temporalis muscle and the consequent temporal hollow?

DR. MCKINNON

There is a potential problem of temporal hollow in shallowness after any use of part or all of the muscle. Using part of the muscle spares some of that problem, and transposition of the posterior two-thirds of the muscle anteriorly, as was done, is also important to minimize the temporal hollow. I don't know what effect radiation therapy had on the patient's growth from the age she started until the postoperative 3-year result. If hollowness persists, as there is to some degree in this case, it can be further improved by a turnover of the remaining portion of the temporal aponeurosis and fascia or a turnover of the muscle itself into the shallowest portion of the temporal hollow.

A question also asked was, why not use only the fascia/aponeurosis flap? The blood supply of the fascial flap is dependent on the superficial temporal artery, contrasted to the deep branches of the maxillary artery that supply the muscle or aponeurosis.

A second reason is because the muscle can be readvanced in the case of flap death; that's a lifeboat. Finally, although the length of the fascial flap would have been sufficient since it approximates the length that was necessary in this sturdier case, I felt that the pericranium provided a cover for the prosthesis that was to be used immediately.

DR. ELLIOT

This reconstruction in this area is managed with a temporalis muscle or temporalis fascia flap, but it is often good to look elsewhere to bring in well-vascularized tissue that doesn't rob from the adjacent area that is already affected by tumor, resection, and radiation. Three flap choices for reconstruction in this area might include muscle flaps, skin flaps, or fat flap, such as omentum. In fact, the latter free flap choice of omentum probably is better than a muscle flap, which might be more traditionally elected because of the fact of atrophy and the predictability of its size. One of the things seen in this patient is a change over time with a gradual retruded appearance of the orbit. Another choice in this case might be a scapular fascial flap or a superficial inferior epigastric artery flap from the abdomen that would bring fat that you can count on for its predictability in its size as the patient grew.

Dr. Toth

I don't see any role for free tissue transfer in a case such as this where there has been no previous surgical violation of anatomy. Nor do I see the need for removal of muscle when the temporoparietal fascia would have done everything that was needed in this reconstruction. There was no reason to suspect potential clotting of the superficial temporal system secondary to radiation—this could be easily verified by direct palpation or by Doppler. You could have extended your superficial temporal fascia to the apex of the skull, which would have given you more than adequate tissue to wrap around your prosthesis and probably, more importantly, would have allowed you to leave your temporalis muscle for the potential of secondary reconstruction. This would have allowed the potential of bringing the temporal muscle in as a secondary reconstruction, either alone or with bone, if necessary, and you would not have burned that potential bridge.

Dr. Grotting

The anatomy of this area has been studied in great detail by a number of different authors. Dr. Rafael Cassanova did a beautiful study of this area, demonstrating that there were, in fact, a variety of tissue planes that were vascularized by various systems. I think it was clear from those studies that when you elevate the true fascia of the temporalis muscle you find yourself in a virtually bloodless plane. In fact, the blood supply to the pericranium, which Dr. Cassanova termed the "innominate fascia," is simply the extension of the pericranium over the temporalis aponeurosis. The blood supply to this particular anatomic layer comes not from the temporalis muscle but rather from a branch of the middle temporal artery, not the deep temporal vessels that supply the muscle. Although the pericranium can be taken as an extension of the temporalis muscle, I do not believe that the temporalis muscle is providing the major blood supply to the pericranium.

I think the choice of the procedure here was a good one and I would agree that free tissue transfer in this situation would have involved more surgery than was required. I have also seen this type of problem handled with a contralateral forehead flap based on the supratrochlear vessels from the opposite side simply turned in to reline the orbit. I think this is a very simple solution, providing skin and some additional fat and soft tissue to support the prosthesis.

DR. ZUBOWICZ

The anatomy that Dr. Grotting described notwithstanding, the operation does work with or without bone. I have used bone on traumatic cases and it does quite nicely. Whether or not it is getting direct nourishment from the temporal muscle, or whether the muscle is providing a vascular bed with the bone graft, or the bone effectively functions as a bone graft, was irrelevant because it did not solve the problem. I don't think one should necessarily shun that approach based on anatomy.

The second point is that a hollow can sometimes result when the temporalis is used. That has happened to me on several occasions and, in those circumstances, I have used a small piece of Proplast custom carved and it seems to work well.

DR. TOTH

Why make the treatment as bad as the disease itself? I can't entertain a forehead flap, leaving a forehead scar, to reconstruct the orbit when we have at our disposal the potential of harvesting a well-vascularized flap based on the superficial temporal muscle that will allow for no direct visible morbidity and will provide the type of coverage necessary within the orbit.

When one is raising the temporoparietal fascia, one should raise the flap at the beginning of the procedure when the scalp is under its resting tension. You can approach the flap directly through the same coronal incision, but extend your coronal incision only down to the level just beneath the hair follicle, plot out the anterior branch of the superficial temporal artery, and stay in the plane directly below the hair follicles, and then deepen the dissection to the plane above the pericranium. Then dissect back proximally to the superficial temporal vessels.

Dr. McKinnon

Let me take a moment to respond. The experience in Atlanta and elsewhere has been more towards the use of free flaps for a situation such as this patient's. I think that this case still demonstrates the utility of the temporal muscle for orbital reconstruction. Far too often this type of orbital exenteration has been reconstructed with a bulky flap that will ultimately be covered by a black patch. By using the temporal muscle and its "system" of contiguous fascia, aponeurosis, and pericranium, a simple, immediate reconstruction of thin tissue has allowed for primary healing and a permanent prosthesis to be worn. Lid sparing, as was done here, would also have been worthless had a bulky flap been placed within the orbital cavity.

2

DECISION MAKING
IN
BREAST
RECONSTRUCTION

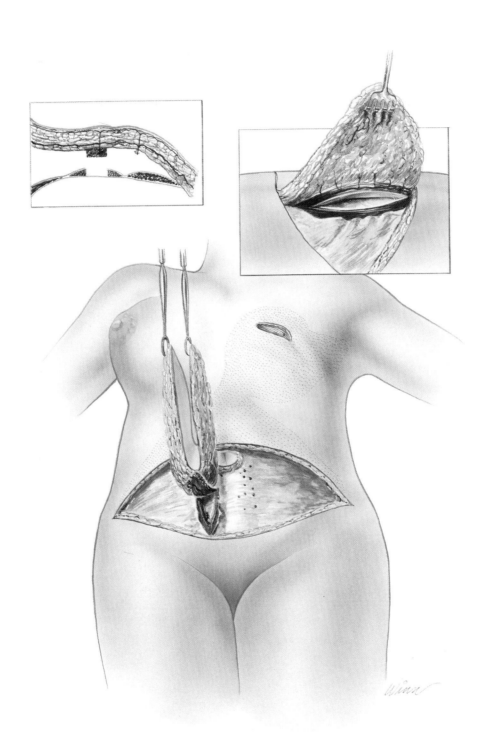

CRITICAL CHOICES IN BREAST RECONSTRUCTION

BRYANT A. TOTH AND BRYAN G. FORLEY

INTRODUCTION

The diagnosis of breast cancer combines the trauma of managing a potentially fatal disease with a radical assault on the body image of the patient. Women afflicted with this disease in the 1990s are bombarded with a multitude of choices regarding both treatment and reconstructive options at an extremely vulnerable and anxious time in their lives. Complicating the decision is the inevitable disagreement among physicians as to the best modality for surgical treatment and/or the need for adjunctive radiation or chemotherapy. The additional option of breast reconstruction compounds the choices faced by the patient, her general surgeon, and her plastic surgeon.

The decision between synthetic implant and autogenous tissue is made more difficult by the issue of immediate or delayed reconstruction. The plastic surgeon must educate the patient and general surgeons about the different alternatives available and their relative advantages and disadvantages. A good cancer operation should be discussed within the context of the patient's reconstructive potential. The key element in surgical decision making is to tailor the procedures more closely to the exact reconstructive needs of each individual patient.

THE PROBLEM

The patient is a 51-year-old woman who underwent right breast lumpectomy and radiation to treat an infiltrating ductal carcinoma. The treatment left her with a breast that appeared distorted with a laterally displaced nipple–areola complex (Figure 4.1a-b). She presented with a new primary carcinoma in her left breast (lobular carcinoma in situ) and a modified radical mastectomy was planned. The patient wanted to have the mastectomy as soon as possible, with reconstruction of both breasts. A bilateral transverse rectus abdominis myocutaneous (TRAM) flap was selected. However, the patient expressed concern about the demands of immediate reconstruction, with time lost from work and the need for blood availability. The procedure was adapted to her particular requirements for bilateral reconstruction with one previously irradiated breast.

The patient underwent a left skin-sparing mastectomy using the modified Wise (inverted "T") pattern skin excision. A total submuscular textured tissue expander was placed at the time of her initial surgery. The use of the expander enabled the preservation and expansion of her skin envelope until such time as the autogenous tissue reconstruction could be per-

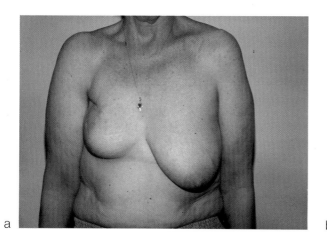
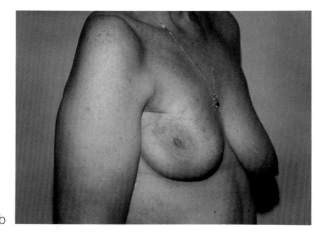

a

b

Figure 4.1.(a,b). This 51-year-old woman underwent right breast lumpectomy and radiation to treat an infiltrating ductal carcinoma. The treatment resulted in a distorted-appearing breast with a laterally displaced nipple–areola complex.

Figure 4.2. A new primary carcinoma in the patient's left breast was found (lobular carcinoma in situ). The patient underwent a skin-sparing modified radical mastectomy using the modified Wise (inverted "T") pattern skin excision. Autogenous tissue reconstruction was desired by the patient but not at the time of the initial surgery. A total submuscular textured tissue expander was placed to enable preservation and expansion of her skin envelope until such time as the autogenous tissue reconstruction could be performed.

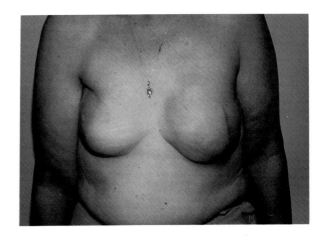

formed (Figure 4.2). This procedure would allow for complete coverage of the deepithelialized TRAM flap. The patchlike effect that would result from fitting the flap to a skin-deficient chest was thereby avoided. An expander was not placed in the remaining right breast because of the prior radiation.

A second operation was planned to accommodate the busy schedule of the patient. She underwent a bilateral TRAM reconstruction with a completion mastectomy of the right breast. The flap was deepithelialized and covered by the expanded skin of the left breast. The right breast demonstrates the patchlike effect that results from conventional techniques that require use of the cutaneous portion of the flap due to inadequate breast skin availability (Figure 4.3a-c). A third procedure was performed to reconstruct both nipple–areola complexes.

TREATMENT OPTIONS

The preceding case is presented to illustrate the versatility of various reconstructive modalities when applied to a challenging patient. It demonstrates the need to customize the operation to each patient and not to rely on a routine approach when reconstructing the breast. The techniques we utilized in this patient will be described within the context of our overall approach to breast reconstruction.

Figure 4.3.(a-c). Following complete mastectomy of the right breast, a bilateral TRAM reconstruction was performed. The expanded skin of the left breast was used to cover the deepithelialized ipsilateral portion of the flap. The patchlike effect that results from use of the cutaneous portion of the flap because of inadequate availability of breast skin is demonstrated in the right breast.

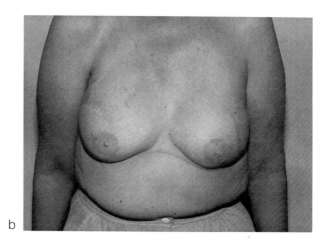

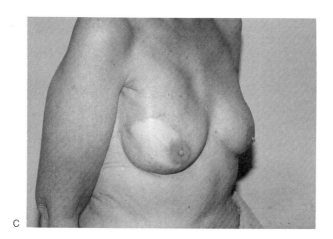

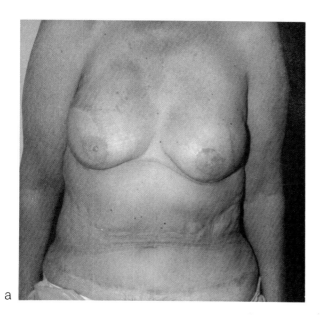

Once the patient has been diagnosed with breast cancer, her first treating physician will usually be her general surgeon. This surgeon acts as the gatekeeper in informing the patient as to the reconstructive options. Today improved patient awareness often results in the patient initiating the discussion of reconstruction with the general surgeon. A good working relationship with the general surgeon, therefore, is essential in optimizing the reconstructive result.

The trend toward lumpectomy and radiation is based on the concept of preservation of an aesthetic and functional breast. In general, we would like to avoid more extensive resections when they do not improve the long-term survival. Unfortunately, with lumpectomy and radiation therapy we occasionally see deformed "preserved" breasts that are aesthetically inferior to those that could be offered with reconstructive techniques. The final appearance of the reconstructed breast is greatly dependent on the relative amounts of skin and breast tissue excised at the time of the mastectomy and on the exact location of the skin incision.

If a formal modified radical mastectomy is judged to be the therapeutic option of choice, the traditional wide ellipse of skin taken with the breast should be reconsidered. Breast cancer is a malignancy of the glandular breast and is now widely believed to be a systemic disease in its earliest stages.[1] In disease that is not locally advanced, it has been found that the skin excision does not impact on overall survival rates. Microscopic disease is better treated by radiation therapy than by more extensive surgical procedures.[2]

In conjunction with our general surgery colleagues, we have been using modified skin incisions[3] that allow the performance of complete mastectomy without sacrificing unnecessary breast skin (Figure 4.4). The nipple-areola complex and the biopsy site are always included in the specimen, and a noncontinuous incision may be added for access to the axillary contents. These skin-sparing incisions vary based on the exact location of the tumor and the size of the breast. It is important to remember that incisions, not excisions, provide the exposure necessary to perform a mastectomy.

Each patient presents an individual problem in breast reconstruction for which an individualized solution must be sought. Generalizations about our approach can only be made if we separately consider the reconstructive demands faced in a small-breasted versus a large-breasted woman. Each reconstructive modality produces a breast that differs in its shape, projection, and ptosis. Each procedure has different risks, recovery periods, and costs. These factors must be considered along with the type and location of the tumor, age, family history, prior surgery, smoking history, plans for childbearing, body habits, lifestyle, and personality when evaluating each reconstructive candidate.

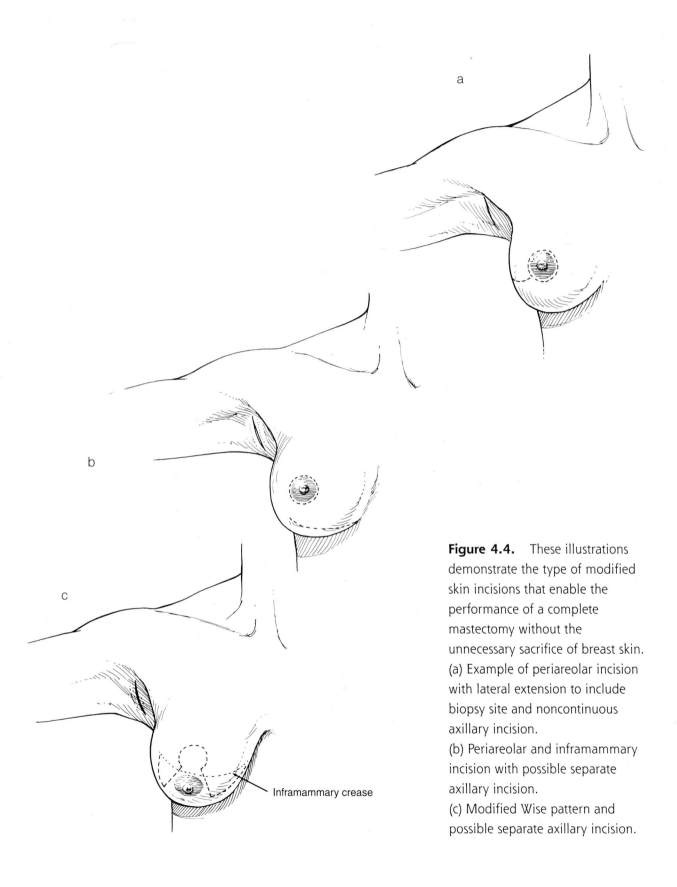

Figure 4.4. These illustrations demonstrate the type of modified skin incisions that enable the performance of a complete mastectomy without the unnecessary sacrifice of breast skin.
(a) Example of periareolar incision with lateral extension to include biopsy site and noncontinuous axillary incision.
(b) Periareolar and inframammary incision with possible separate axillary incision.
(c) Modified Wise pattern and possible separate axillary incision.

Inframammary crease

SMALL-BREASTED PATIENT

The small-breasted patient is often thin and has nonptotic breasts that may be the easiest to reconstruct in terms of matching the uninvolved breast. However, they are also subject to potential pitfalls such as decreased breast projection due to contracture of the surgical scars. The initial biopsy is best performed via a periareolar incision. A horizontal or oblique biopsy scar can result in decreased breast projection when the general surgeon performs a traditional mastectomy with a skin ellipse excision that includes the scar. Wound contraction that results in decreased projection can be minimized if the mastectomy incision is made noncontinuous with the biopsy site scar. The need for additional exposure can be met with an additional incision in the inframammary fold or a separate incision for axillary dissection.

Thus, in the small-breasted woman, the outcome of reconstruction will be enhanced when the mastectomy is performed by a periareolar incision, combined with an inframammary fold incision if necessary, and a separate axillary crease incision for the axillary dissection. A good alternative for slightly larger breasts is a modified Wise (inverted "T") pattern skin excision. Both of these excisions will avoid transverse scars across the apex of the breast mound that would inhibit final projection.

The nonptotic, small, youthful breast can be readily matched in two stages using a tissue expander followed by placement of a permanent implant. A single-stage placement of an implant in a patient undergoing immediate reconstruction can lead to unpredictable results. The use of an expander allows the reconstructive surgeon increased control over the final skin envelope and a choice of the best implant position. In immediate reconstruction, total submuscular placement of the implant is necessary to prevent suluxation into the axillary dissection and to provide cover for the implant in the event of skin wound problems. Adequate pocket dissection inferiorly will minimize the risk of superior breast fullness. Special attention is paid to the medial and lateral extent of the dissection and to the location of the inframammary fold to precisely match the contralateral breast.

Many of these same concerns arise in the patient undergoing delayed reconstruction. These patients often require a longer period of expansion than patients undergoing immediate reconstruction because of scar formation and skin retraction. Total muscular cover is not mandatory in patients with a delayed reconstruction.

There are multiple considerations in the choice of implant for the patient with small, nonptotic breasts. A permanent prosthesis with a remote port that is removable on a delayed basis (such as the Siltex Spectrum) allows a single-stage mound reconstruction. If a two-stage procedure is chosen, a textured tissue expander is placed either at the time of the mastectomy or at a later date. After the tissue has been expanded to 20% to 30% beyond the volume of the opposite breast, the expander is replaced with a textured gel or saline permanent implant. We believe that silicone gel provides a more natural-feeling breast than do saline implants, but their use is clouded by safety issues and new governmental regulations. The ultimate choice of implant is based on patient preference after a thorough explanation of all safety concerns and potential complications.

The nonptotic small-breasted patient is also a good candidate for reconstruction with autogenous tissue. The natural tendency toward ptosis of the autogenous tissue can be adjusted by paying special attention to the relative area of the skin envelope compared to the volume of tissue replacement. The ptotic small-breasted patient may require a mastopexy on the contralateral breast. This should be performed at a later stage, with adequate time (a minimum of 3 months) allowed for the reconstructed breast to achieve its final form.

The contralateral unipedicle TRAM flap, as developed by Hartrampf,[4] is the procedure of choice for autogenous tissue, but may be inadequate in the thin patient who has medium-sized breasts. The pedicle is reliable and the results are predictable, except for occasional fat necrosis. We prefer the use of a skin-sparing mastectomy in combination with the deepithelialized TRAM flap for volume to reconstruct a natural-appearing breast with an intact skin envelope of normal color and texture. The preservation of the breast skin avoids the patchlike effect that results from fitting the abdominal skin into the breast defect created after traditional mastectomy elliptical skin excisions. We have found minimal morbidity with the TRAM flap in the average patient.

Microvascular transfer of the TRAM flap is indicated in the younger patient who is concerned about abdominal wall functional impairment. Smoking, a requirement for all of the available abdominal wall tissue of the reconstruction, and prior abdominal wall incisions such as for a cholecystectomy are also indications for microvascular techniques. The patient who has future plans for childbearing must be counseled as to the potential problems if a TRAM flap is used for breast reconstruction.

LARGE-BREASTED PATIENT

Reconstruction of the patient with large breasts often requires matching a large and ptotic opposite breast. The reconstructive priorities of the patient should be discussed preoperatively and should include the option of a mastopexy or reduction procedure on the opposite breast.

The aesthetic result in the large-breasted patient is greatly enhanced with the use of skin-sparing mastectomy incisions. Projection of the reconstructed breast is best preserved with use of a modified Wise (inverted "T") pattern skin excision for the mastectomy. A separate incision may be used, if necessary, to excise the biopsy site or for the axillary dissection.

Reconstruction of a large breast with a prosthesis should always be performed in a two-stage procedure with an expander. Most attempts to match the opposite large breast in a single stage with a fixed prosthesis will be marred by postoperative capsular contracture. A textured expander such as the McGhan "Biocell" provides good projection in the large breast, though with some superior fullness.

As in the small-breasted patient, total submuscular placement of the expander must be used in patients undergoing immediate reconstruction. In the delayed setting, subtotal muscular coverage is acceptable. The exact permanent implants to be used are selected after discussion of the relative safety issues with the patient. We often use the technique of stacking the textured implants to achieve greater projection of the reconstructed breast. We generally find that the best position for the stacked implants is with the smaller device placed anterior to the larger prosthesis. Symmetry is the greatest problem in the large-breasted patient, because of the difficulty of matching the opposite ptotic breast with implants.

The use of autogenous tissue to reconstruct a large breast is more problematic than in the small-breasted patient because of the large volume that is required. These patients are frequently older and must be carefully scrutinized as to their medical suitability for this more demanding reconstructive procedure. The TRAM flap is still our technique of choice to match the large opposite breast. However, one must be sure that the blood supply is adequate to support the volume of tissue needed to match the opposite breast. Ischemia can result in fat necrosis and partial or total skin loss. This occurs more frequently in older, fatter patients than in younger, thinner patients.

The bipedicle technique is often used in unilateral breast reconstruction to assure the survival of the random portion of the TRAM flap (zone 4 as defined by Hartrampf) or in the patient with limited abdominal tissue compared to breast size. Greater reconstructive versatility is provided by splitting the two hemi-abdominal TRAM flaps based on their individual muscular pedicles. The two portions of the flap can then be stacked or layered to reconstruct chest wall contour defects in addition to providing better projection and volume.

The deformity that results from a radical mastectomy will always require additional tissue to recreate the anterior axillary fold and to fill the infraclavicular defect. If the patient so desires, the autogenous tissue technique can be combined with implants for greater volume. Microvascular transplant of the TRAM flap, in the previously operated abdomen, can be used to spare the morbidity of bilateral loss of the rectus muscles or to increase blood supply in the obese patient, the smoker, or the diabetic.

TECHNIQUES OF RECONSTRUCTION

Expander and Implant

Tissue expanders for patients undergoing immediate reconstruction must be totally covered by muscle. Submuscular placement will prevent the implant from migrating superiorly or from subluxation into the axilla. Preoperative markings of the native inframammary fold on both sides and planned skin incisions are made in the upright position. The general surgeon must avoid injury to the serratus and pectoralis muscles during the mastectomy to minimize problems with expander cover. If oncologically appropriate, the fascia should be preserved. Delayed reconstruction does not require total coverage of the expander except in very trim patients. The pectoralis major can be approached from its inferior margin and a pocket developed that may have a partial subcutaneous component inferiorly.

The simplest technique to develop a total submuscular pocket is to incise the serratus muscle directly over a rib in the inferior aspect of the pocket close to the inframammary fold. The pocket is developed by dissecting the serratus fibers from the ribs using the fiberoptic electrocautery unit (Figure 4.5a-b). A plane is created between the serratus anterior and the ribs and intercostal muscles. The pocket is developed as far medially as possible without detaching the pectoralis origin or parasternal perforators. The inferior dissection is continued to approximately one fingerbreadth below the planned inframammary fold. The dissection extends to the anterior axillary line laterally and to approximately the second rib superiorly (Figure 4.6).

The textured expanders and implants allow precise positioning at the level of the inframammary fold. Assuming uneventful skin healing, expansion is begun 10 days postoperatively and repeated every 7 to 10 days until the size exceeds that of the uninvolved breast by 20% to 30%. The permanent implant is placed by incising directly through the pectoralis muscle and closing the wound in layers. Complete capsulectomy is not re-

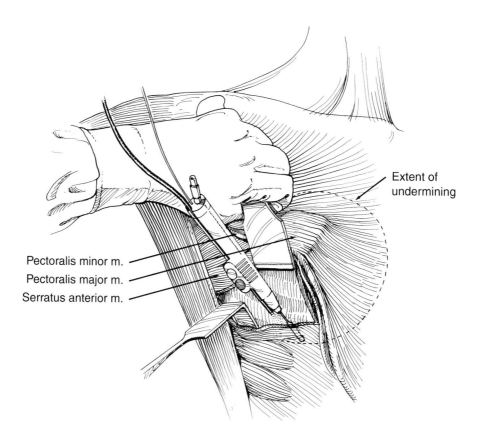

Pectoralis minor m.
Pectoralis major m.
Serratus anterior m.

Extent of
undermining

Figure 4.5.(a). Submuscular dissection of the serratus anterior muscle to develop the inferolateral portion of the pocket for tissue expander placement is performed using the fiberoptic electrocautery unit. This muscle is very adherent to the ribs and care must be taken to maintain pocket integrity.

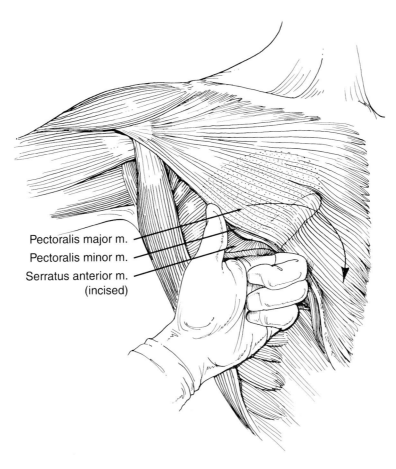

Pectoralis major m.
Pectoralis minor m.
Serratus anterior m.
(incised)

Figure 4.5.(b). The superomedial portion of the pocket can usually be developed with blunt finger dissection underneath the pectoralis major.

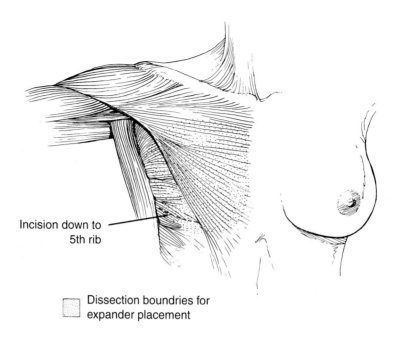

Incision down to
5th rib

Dissection boundries for
expander placement

Figure 4.6. The dissection boundaries for expander placement are shown superimposed over anatomic landmarks: superiorly to the second rib, inferiorly to 2 cm below the inframammary fold, laterally to the anterior axillary line, and medially to the pectoralis major origin.

quired at the time of implant exchange when a textured expander is utilized. This procedure is frequently done on an outpatient basis.

TRAM Flap

The TRAM flap can be performed synchronously with the mastectomy in the patient undergoing immediate reconstruction. Preoperative markings of the breast and abdomen are performed in the upright position (Figure 4.7). The umbilicus is circumferentially incised through the skin with the scalpel and then dissected to its stalk with the Metzenbaum scissors. The upper margin of the planned elliptical skin island is incised superior to the umbilicus extending to the level of the anterior superior iliac spine. An incision at the suprapubic crease extending to the lateral extent of the upper incision is used as the inferior margin of the skin island. The fascial perforators are preserved by beveling the fat incisions away from the skin flaps.

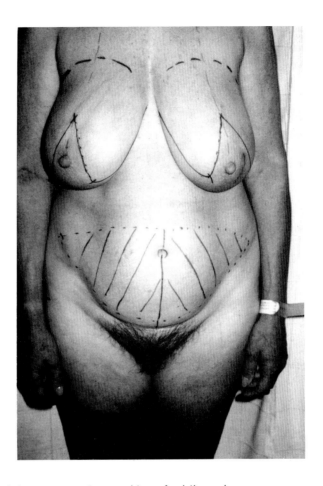

Figure 4.7. Illustration of the preoperative markings for bilateral reconstruction using the TRAM flap. The modified Wise pattern skin excision is to be used in this case to preserve sufficient skin to allow for complete coverage of the deepithelialized TRAM flap.

The dissection is extended to the anterior abdominal wall fascia and carried superiorly to the costal margins.

A vertical incision is then made in the anterior rectus fascia at approximately the midpoint of each muscle down to the level of the abdominal flap. The fascia is then elevated to the lateral border of the rectus muscle and medially to the linea alba. The abdominal flap is elevated from the abdominal wall fascia laterally to the level of the periumbilical perforators. If a bipedicle flap or bilateral reconstruction is planned, the mirror-image perforators are preserved on both sides of the umbilicus (Figure 4.8).

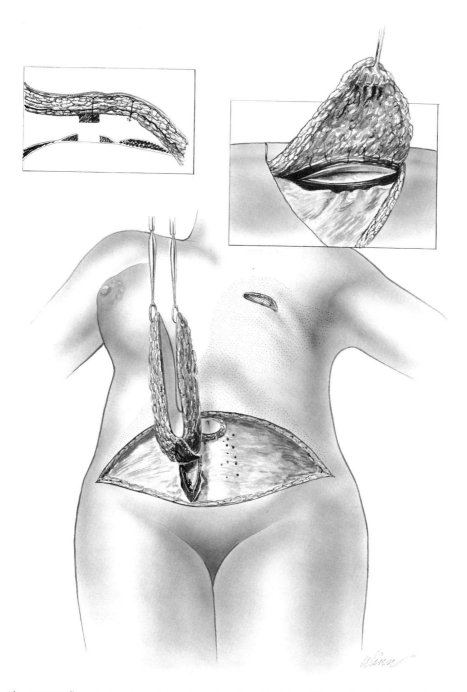

Figure 4.8. The TRAM flap is developed by elevating the skin island from the abdominal wall fascia laterally to the level of the periumbilical perforators. The anterior rectus fascia is incised and a cuff of rectus abdominus muscle lateral to the epigastric vessels and periumbilical perforators is preserved from the costal margin to the arcuate line. A 1.0-cm strip of muscle is also preserved medially for support in abdominal closure. An anterior rectus fascial cuff remains attached to the muscle and is incised to include the periumbilical perforators.

A muscle-splitting incision is used to preserve a cuff of muscle from the costal margin to the arcuate line lateral to the epigastric vessels and periumbilical perforators. A strip of muscle approximately 1.0 cm wide is preserved medially to add to the support system of the abdomen in the closure. The anterior rectus fascia is preserved between the flap and the muscle in the area of the periumbilical perforators. The rectus muscle is then inferiorly divided just below the arcuate line after further dissection and ligation of the inferior epigastric vessels. The dissection of the entire rectus muscle flap from the intact posterior rectus fascia is continued to the level of the costal cartilages. The flap is then passed through an inferomedial subcutaneous tunnel into the area of the chest defect (Figure 4.9a-b). Care is taken not to twist the pedicle or to allow tension. The rectus muscle can be partially divided laterally at the lateral costal margin to increase its arc of rotation and to decrease tension.

The anterior rectus fascial incision is completely closed with two layers of continuous, double-stranded, 0-nylon sutures incorporating the medial and lateral cuffs of rectus muscle. Gradual tightening of the suture distributes forces along the suture line. In both unilateral and bilateral rectus muscle procedures, wide approximation of the lateral abdominal wall fascia is performed to reinforce the closure (Figure 4.10a-b). This closure technique, adapted from Hartrampf, utilizes two separate 0-nylon sutures, which are simultaneously criss-crossed starting inferiorly to the superior extent of the fascial closure. Marlex mesh is rarely necessary to strengthen the abdominal wall.

Closure of the abdomen is preceded by location of the new umbilicus. Tension on the umbilicus can result in necrosis because of its poor vascularity. 3-0 Vicryl suture is used to suture the fascia at the base of the umbilical stalk to the dermis of the abdominal skin to avoid tension on the umbilicus. The skin edges of the umbilicus are then sutured with plain gut to the abdominal skin. The abdomen is closed in three layers with the placement of two suction drains. The midline is always the tightest part of the closure. A less strangulated closure can be achieved by starting with a suprapubic "W" incision. The upper abdominal flap edge is longer than

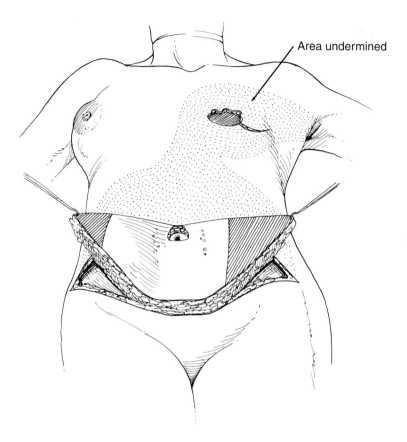

Figure 4.9.(a). This illustration demonstrates the completed dissection of the unipedicle flap with the poorly perfused zones 3 and 4 marked for discard. The subcutaneous tunnel into the chest wall defect is shown.

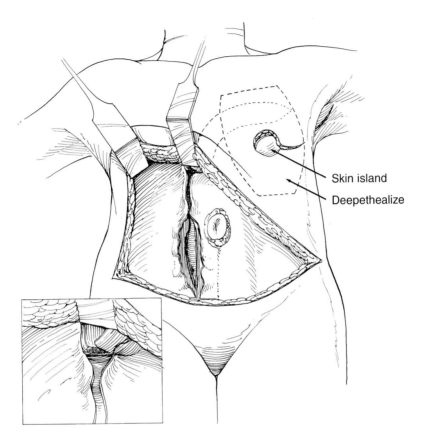

Skin island

Deepethealize

Figure 4.9.(b). Passage of the flap into the chest defect is often facilitated by a partial lateral division of the rectus muscle to increase the arc of rotation.

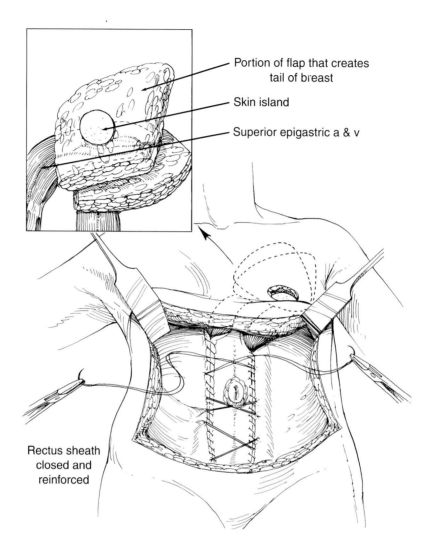

Portion of flap that creates
tail of breast

Skin island

Superior epigastric a & v

Rectus sheath
closed and
reinforced

Figure 4.10.(a). A split bilateral TRAM flap is used in this illustration to reconstruct a unilateral chest wall defect. Splitting the flap enables greater versatility to create projection of the breast and to improve contour defects. The abdomen is closed with two layers of continuous double-stranded 0-nylon sutures incorporating the remaining medial and lateral cuffs of rectus muscle. Wide closure, which includes both defects, is then begun inferiorly with two alternating sutures. Care is taken not to strangulate the pedicles.

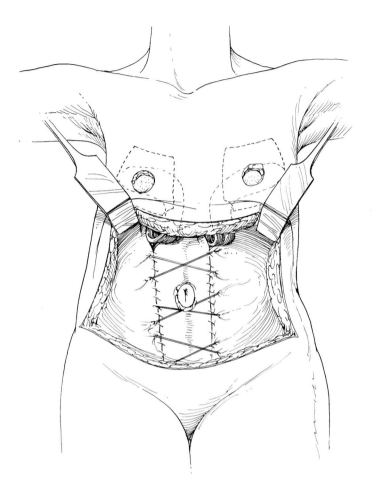

Figure 4.10.(b). Reconstruction of a bilateral chest wall defect is shown with a wide fascial closure used to reinforce the abdominal wall.

the lower edge, so closure should always be lateral-to-medial to decrease redundant areas of skin and to leave the "dog-ears" centrally rather than laterally.

The flap is tailored to match the opposite breast. Better definition of the inframammary fold can be achieved by suturing the deepithelialized dermis of the lower edge of the flap to the chest wall. If skin-sparing techniques are utilized with a modified Wise pattern, the only exposed flap skin will be in the circular defect from the nipple–areola excision.

CONCLUSIONS

The techniques of breast reconstruction have expanded beyond that of simply augmenting the chest wall. Reconstruction should no longer be regarded as an afterthought to be considered once the disease process has been treated. The present-day reconstructive surgeon must be dedicated to achieving the most natural-appearing breast by tailoring the available techniques to match the needs of the individual patient. This necessitates early involvement of the patient to discuss the available options and ascertain her desires. A treatment and reconstructive plan is then coordinated with the general surgeon to achieve the optimum result for each patient.

ROUNDTABLE DISCUSSION

DR. TOTH

Each patient for breast reconstruction provides a separate, individualized challenge. In the case example that we have presented we elected to blend tissue expansion with autologous-tissue reconstruction in an attempt to spare skin and minimize scarring. These are not the obvious solutions for every problem, but in this particular patient it worked out well. Certainly this patient could have been approached in a variety of other ways with an equally satisfactory result.

DR. MOSES

While this patient has a beautiful result, it seems to me that it breaks one of the cardinal tenets of bilateral breast reconstruction, which is to do the same thing on both sides. Since you are going to have a patch of abdominal skin on one side, why not do the same thing and have a patch of abdominal skin on both sides so that you can at least get symmetry.

DR. TOTH

In breast reconstruction when one side is immediate and the other side delayed, it is often very difficult to create the same problem. You have scarred, irradiated skin on the right side, and on the left side you have fresh nonirradiated tissue. It's no different from matching an existing breast with a single reconstructed breast.

DR. ELLIOTT

I agree with Dr. Toth that these are two different breasts from the start and they are always going to be two different breasts, but I think that we can achieve symmetry, as he has shown beautifully in this patient. The timing of surgery for this patient influenced her choices. I think that just doing the mastectomy and coming back with the bilateral TRAM flaps later might have been just as good. I realize that the expander was inserted to maintain the skin envelope, but I'm not sure how important that is. It seems to me that the bilateral TRAM could just have been done secondarily.

DR. STAHL

I think that in patients with large, pendulous breasts, it seems like a good idea to use a Wise pattern incision, although certainly not in everyone. It also seems that you advocate the use of an expander in almost every implant reconstruction: is that correct?

DR. TOTH

That is correct; I don't ever use just an implant. In those cases where I may be able to match the remaining breast with an implant, I use an adjustable implant like the Siltex Spectrum type of expander. It's nice to be able to have the additional contour without any greater morbidity. The adjustable expander allows you additional flexibility in terms of being able to overexpand and then withdraw fluid with the small price of needing to have the port removed at a later time.

DR. MOSES

We plastic surgeons are used to the Wise pattern when we approach patients for breast reduction and we all have our idiosyncratic ways of marking these patients. Explain how you approach the marking of a large-breasted patient for a mastectomy using the Wise pattern: where the measurements are, where the limbs are, and how the markings might differ from the standard markings for a breast-reduction patient.

DR. TOTH

In this patient, the ultimate location of the nipple–areolar complex did not end up on the apex of the "T". I do not commit myself to the ultimate location of the nipple–areolar complex, and I use the "T" incisions to avoid scarring in the superior hemisphere of the breast. The attractiveness of this type of incision is that the patient can wear a low-cut dress with a low decolletage and not have scars that are directly visible. With regard to marking, I try to leave as much skin as possible, with a low threshold for removing additional skin after the mastectomy. I am constantly concerned about the potential for traction injury on the skin tips and flaps at the time the mastectomy is done, so I leave all of this tissue and then I can trim it in the future.

DR. STAHL

For the last couple of years, I have been doing the modified Lassus reduction in our reduction mammoplasty patients. We might think about trying to use the more limited vertical scar in select mastectomy patients too.

You also mentioned subluxation of the implant into the axilla. Are you really having difficulty with this? I haven't had this problem as long as we recognize where the extent of the mastectomy dissection has been. The greater use of textured implants has made this less of a problem as well.

Dr. Toth

It's not a problem as long as there is total muscular coverage of your expander. Certainly the implant would have a tendency to migrate into the axilla if it were only in a subcutaneous pocket.

Dr. Grotting

This case brings up a number of interesting issues. I was interested in your persistence with the concept of overexpansion. The original concept was that you could actually produce some ptosis by overexpansion and then dropping back. In my opinion this has not really worked out. My practice is simply to expand to the level that you need. Rather than overexpansion, I think that additional time for the softening of the soft tissues over the expander has been responsible for a more natural skin envelope.

I think that placing an expander in anticipation of replacing it with autogenous tissue is a good idea, but the ideal time to place autogenous tissue and to prevent the contraction of the skin envelope would be at the time of the initial mastectomy. I understand that in this particular case there were timing issues involved that made you select this particular course of action. If your intent is to transfer the autogenous tissue in the future as a free-tissue transfer, keep in mind the state of the recipient vessels. In terms of scarring of the recipient vessels, the ideal time to transfer the autogenous tissue would be at the time of the mastectomy. This can be done without blood transfusions.

I think the issue of the abdominal donor site needs to be carefully examined. Many surgeons who have been doing TRAM flaps are reporting an increasing incidence of hernia as time goes by. They are also recognizing increased weakness of the abdominal wall in individuals who have had both rectus muscles removed. I think that the trend toward using both rectus muscles simply in the interest of increasing blood supply to the TRAM flap territory is one that should be discouraged. Understandably, not everyone is interested in and/or capable of transferring the lower abdominal skin island as a free-tissue transfer, but we should note that the primary blood supply to the lower abdominal skin island comes through the inferior epigastric system. When the TRAM flap can be transferred as a free-tissue transfer, both preservation of abdominal wall function and preservation of the aesthetics of the reconstructed breast can be improved.

Dr. Toth

As we critically look at the reconstructed breast, particularly with implants, it is my feeling that where we fail miserably is in dealing with the issue of projection. With overexpansion, I am not looking for an overly expanded pocket, but for expansion in the anterior-posterior direction. It is an attempt to increase projection. In achieving adequate projection you invariably create the appearance of overexpansion in the upper hemisphere.

Your abdominal donor site issues are well taken. Certainly, free-tissue transfer has become an accepted alterative in many types of situations. With this patient's radiation on her right anterior chest wall and axilla, a free-tissue transfer to the thoracodorsal vessels would be more difficult.

Dr. Zubowicz

The problem from a technical side that we have had in cases similar to the one presented is the healing that occurs at the junction of the inverted "T" in the Wise pattern. Fortunately, those wounds, albeit troublesome, generally heal by themselves if the expander is covered by muscle. After the expansion process is complete it is a fairly easy matter to revise those scars, since the expansion process will eventually yield an excess of skin in the first place.

Dr. Elliott

I have also used the Wise pattern for immediate breast reconstruction, but it concerns me more than does a simple transverse skin excision. The chest wall flaps are more reliable and the transverse scar lies just above the inframammary crease. This creates a new skin envelope of the same size as the one resulting from the Wise pattern, but with flaps that are less complicated and safer. Some of the general surgeons who I have worked with will elevate Wise pattern flaps that will be viable and others will yield flaps that won't be safe. For that reason I have returned to transverse excisions. The transverse excision does not allow for the gathering of the skin in the center of the mound, which does contribute to projection. When the nipple goes on in the secondary procedure, you could do a vertical excision of skin, which would be a safer time to give you more projection.

With regard to free flap transfer in the irradiated chest, we have done a number of those and we use as large a vessel as we can find, generally the thoracordorsal trunk. The artery is at least 3.0 mm and the vein is larger. Although we do not enjoy working in an irradiated field, we do not feel that irradiation is a contraindication to free flap transfer.

DR. STAHL

We have heard so much about autologous tissue reconstruction in either current or past smokers. In my experience with rectus flap reconstruction, there have been more problems with ischemia of the mastectomy flaps and the abdominal flaps than with the rectus flap itself. These problems have occurred in the central abdominal closure and, in the large-breasted patient, in the inferomedial mastectomy flap and over the subcutaneous tunnel. I have not, to date, had difficulty with the rectus flap itself.

DR. TOTH

Dr. Elliott, one advantage of the Wise pattern is that it avoids the excess gathering of skin that invariably happens in the axilla after a mastectomy with axillary dissection. Being able to mobilize the skin medially avoids unnecessary gathering, which happens when you do a horizontal excision alone.

DR. MOSES

The Wise pattern excision avoids the tight scar across the apex of the breast and it allows for removal of skin in the side-to-side dimension as well as in the vertical dimension.

DR. GROTTING

I would also recommend caution with the use of the Wise pattern. There is a tendency to compromise the thickness of the skin flaps in an effort to avoid necrosis at the lower end of the "T." Patients are very unhappy with a skin slough.

The problem of lateral axillary skin is easily adjusted at the end of the mastectomy. In immediate breast reconstruction you adjust ptosis and projection by rotating the flap of lateral skin superiorly and medially. This skin should be resected at the time of the initial contouring of the breast mound. The indication for using a Wise pattern, in my mind, is to erase some of the stigmata of breast cancer surgery and breast reconstruction. Obviously, if you do a reduction on the opposite side, you have symmetry of scars. If you don't do anything to the other side, then I think the advantages of the Wise pattern, from the standpoint of psychological rehabilitation of the woman, are less. It is certainly not as safe an incision as the simple lateral incision. Even in patients who are undergoing simple mastectomy or subcutaneous mastectomy, the single lateral incision has been a very acceptable incision from a cosmetic standpoint and it is still easily concealed by most low-cut garments.

DR. TOTH

I am not advocating the Wise incision for every patient. I am advocating that we plastic surgeons be flexible in our approach to our patients and do what is best in each particular situation.

I would like to address Dr. Stahl's question regarding smoking and potential increased morbidity. Although I am concerned about the viability and integrity of the transferred tissue, I am more concerned about potential ischemia of the abdominal skin and inferior flaps of the mastectomy.

DR. STAHL

One thing that compounds the abdominal donor site problem is the proximity of the umbilicus to the location of the abdominal closure scar. The wake of the incision for the umbilical inset seems to be an area of difficulty if it is too close to the donor-site incision. We have to try to plan not only a more lax abdominal closure than usual, but also to place our incision as far away from where the umbilical incision will be.

DR. ELLIOTT

Free TRAMs offer a couple of technical advantages in smokers that should be mentioned. The need for a tunnel is obviated, avoiding the disruption of the xiphoid region perforators, thereby preserving valuable circulation to the abdominal and mastectomy flaps. The abdominal scar can always be made quite low because you are using the inferior perforators. You don't need to move the ellipse up as we would on a superiorly based TRAM flap to increase the flow through the perforators to the flap. Also, the inferior system has better flood flow to the TRAM flap itself, so we are increasingly

using the free TRAM in the past or current smoker who we need to oper-
ate on.

Dr. Grotting

I view the free TRAM technique simply as an alternative way of technically
transferring the lower abdominal tissue. I think that the entire skin island of
the TRAM territory can be safely transferred on the central portion of the
rectus muscle, including the perforators and preserving both the medial and
lateral strips of the intact rectus muscle. The healthier blood supply allows
more initial molding, folding, and plicating of the flap itself.

Dr. McKinnon

What are the oncologic issues of thin skin flaps at the time of the mastectomy?

Dr. Toth

Breast cancer is a parenchymal disease, not a skin disease. Even with a skin-
sparing mastectomy, most recurrences are distant and not local ones. It will
take several decades before we have substantive data showing the incidence
of recurrence in skin-sparing incisions. From my point of view, the mastectomy incisions must include removal of the biopsy site, removal of the breast
parenchyma and nipple–areolar complex, and allow for access to the axilla.
Any type of incision that allows for all of this should be oncologically adequate.

REFERENCES

1. Frykberg ER, Bland KI. Evolution of surgical principles for the management of breast cancer. In: Bland KI, Copeland EM, editors. The Breast: Comprehensive Management of Benign and Malignant Diseases. Philadelphia: Saunders, 1991:539–569.

2. Fisher B, Bauer M, Margolese R, et al. Five-year results of a randomized clinical trial: Comparing total mastectomy and segmental mastectomy with or without radiation in the treatment of breast cancer. N Engl J Med, 1985;312:665.

3. Toth BA, Lappert P. Modified skin incisions for mastectomy: The need for plastic surgical input in preoperative planning. Plast Reconstr Surg, 1991;87:1048.

4. Hartrampf CR Jr. Hartrampf's Breast Reconstruction with Living Tissue. Norfolk, Va.: Hampton Press, 1991.

3
Decision Making
in
Chest
Reconstruction

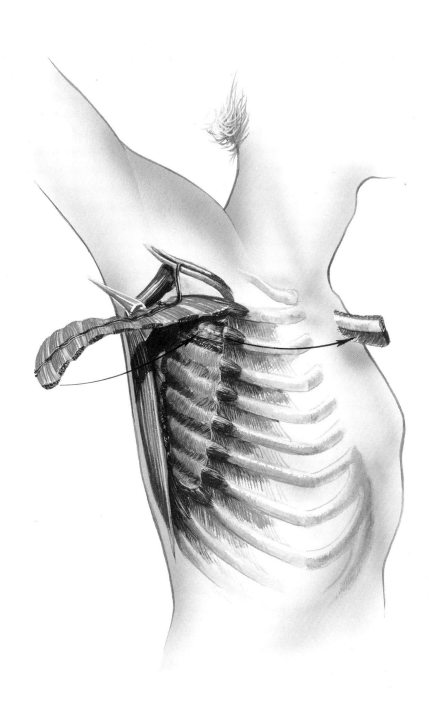

CHEST WALL RECONSTRUCTION: THE STERNAL WOUND

RICHARD S. STAHL AND GARY S. KOPF

THE PROBLEM

A 25-year-old man with Down's syndrome presented with constrictive pericarditis 6 weeks after surgical closure of a ventricular septal defect. Repeat sternotomy was necessitated for pericardiectomy to relieve his constriction.

Two weeks postpericardiectomy, the patient developed signs of sepsis in the setting of a purulent mediastinitis. Cultures ultimately grew *Staphylococcus* (Figures 5.1 and 5.2).

He was stabilized with intravenous antibiotics and operative drainage and debridement. The debridement was followed by a 1-week interval of open-wound care and nutritional supplements. He was then returned to the operating room for complete debridement and definitive closure (Figures 5.3 and 5.4).

The closure was achieved with bilateral pectoralis major muscle flaps, a right rectus abdominus muscle flap, and cutaneous advancement flaps. The right pectoralis flap was a medially based turnover flap used to provide coverage for the midsternal region, the left pectoralis flap was advanced on its thoracoacromial pedicle to primarily address the upper

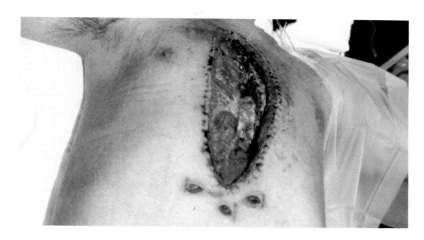

Figure 5.1 and 5.2. This 26-year-old man presented with suppurative mediastinitis following sternectomy for pericardiectomy.

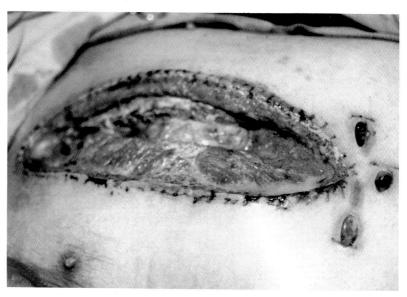

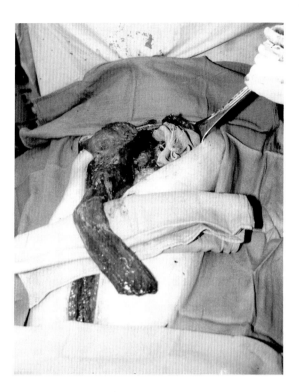

Figure 5.3. After total sternectomy and resection of multiple costal cartilages, three muscle flaps have been elevated to satisfy the defect: one pectoralis turnover flap, one pectoralis advancement flap, and one rectus abdominis flap.

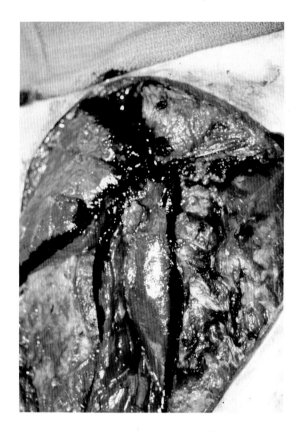

Figure 5.4. The superiorly based rectus abdominis flap is demonstrated. Closure was completed with bilateral cutaneous advancement flaps.

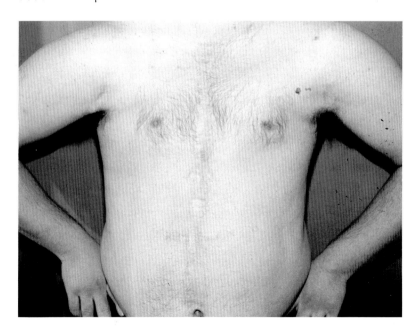

Figure 5.5. The patient is seen in long-term follow-up 8 years later with a well-healed wound.

wound, and the rectus abdominis flap definitively addressed the xiphoid region.

The patient continues to do well after 10 years of follow-up. He is an active athlete (Figure 5.5).

Introduction

Even with low surgical wound complication rates, a significant number of sternal wound complications occur in modern practice owing to the sheer volume of cardiothoracic operations being performed. Most chest wall reconstructive operations are indicated for the treatment of mediastinitis or sternal osteomyelitis. Occasionally, flap coverage is needed to achieve wound closure when conventional closure has resulted in undue cardiac compression. Less commonly, vascularized tissue is needed to obturate chronic mediastinal/intrapericardial or pleural cavities, or buttress or protect complex cardiovascular or tracheobronchial suture lines or patches.

There has been a trend in the treatment of these wounds away from the traditional method of open packing and healing by secondary intention. Healing by secondary intention can be associated with a prolonged, if not stormy, course. If the patient survives the prolonged course, wound healing can result in persistent draining sinus tracts with underlying chondritis or painful, unstable scars lying directly on bone, cartilage, or vital structures.

Historically, continuous antibiotic irrigation techniques were next developed to address these problems.[1,2] They succeeded in many cases, but morbidity and mortality remained higher than desired. Subsequently, Jurkiewicz et al. published a landmark series of infected sternotomy wounds treated with muscle flaps in 1979.[3] This has proven to be the standard against which all other methods of treatment must be measured.

In the 1980s, the hearty pectoralis major flap was firmly entrenched as the workhorse of anterior chest wall reconstruction—especially in the sternotomy wound. Its vascular pattern makes it amenable for use as an advancement flap based on its dominant thoracoacromial pedicle or as a turnover flap based on its internal mammary perforators (Figures 5.6–10).

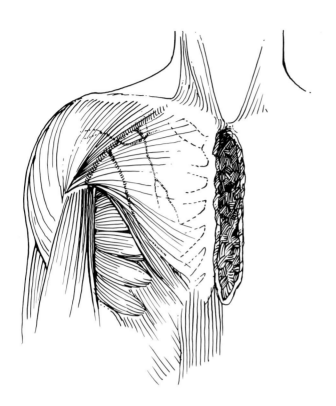

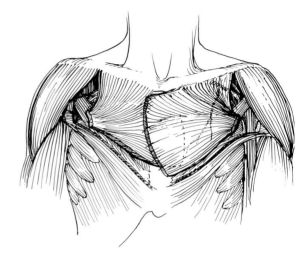

Figure 5.7.

Figure 5.6–5.10. The pectoralis major flap either may be based on the thoracoacromial vessels for advancement medially or it may be turned over based on the internal mammary perforators.

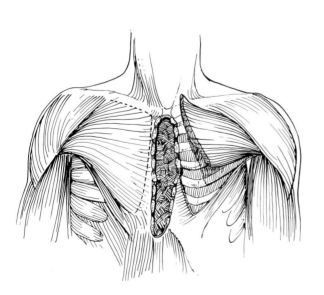

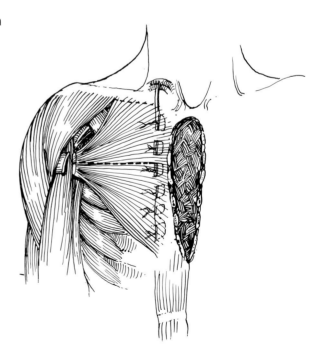

Figure 5.8.

Figure 5.9.

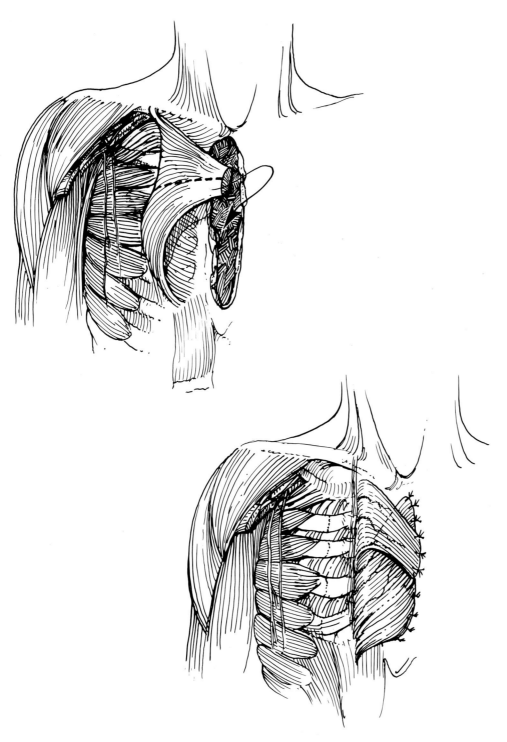

Figure 5.10.

Either way it can be used wholly or in multiple split segments (Figures 5.9, and 5.10). When used as a musculocutaneous advancement flap, it can be readvanced when cardiac or other reoperation is required.

Other pedicled flaps available in the reconstructive armamentarium of the central anterior chest wall include the rectus abdominis, the latissimus dorsi, and the greater omentum (Figures 5.11–13). In addition to these, the serratus anterior, external oblique, trapezius, and paraspinous muscle flaps, the scapular and parascapular flaps, and numerous other named and unnamed fasciocutaneous and cutaneous flaps can be employed for lateral and posterior thoracic reconstruction.

The delivery of a viable muscle flap into a thoracic wound in and of itself will not suffice to cure an established infection, fistula, or other healing problem. Adherence to general principles of surgery, such as aggressive critical care and nutrition, aggressive debridement, obturation of potential spaces, effective hemostasis and suction drainage, and administration of appropriate culture-directed antibiotics, is invaluable in achieving a favorable result.

The following discussion includes an overview of the regional anatomy, with attention to the pectoralis major muscle flap. A section on technique highlights surgical methods of pectoralis muscle flap elevation. The subsequent discussion centers upon the thought processes surrounding appropriate selection of this flap as well as its strengths and weaknesses. Finally, a roundtable discussion concludes the review of this topic.

Anatomy

The pectoralis major is a fan-shaped muscle with multiple origins along the sternocostal junctions and the medial costal surfaces anteromedially and the clavicle superiorly. Its tendinous insertion onto the proximal humerus allows it to adduct and internally rotate the arm.

The dominant blood supply of the pectoralis major is the thoracoacromial artery, which is consistently present along the undersurface of the muscle. The thoracoacromial artery also gives off a branch to the pec-

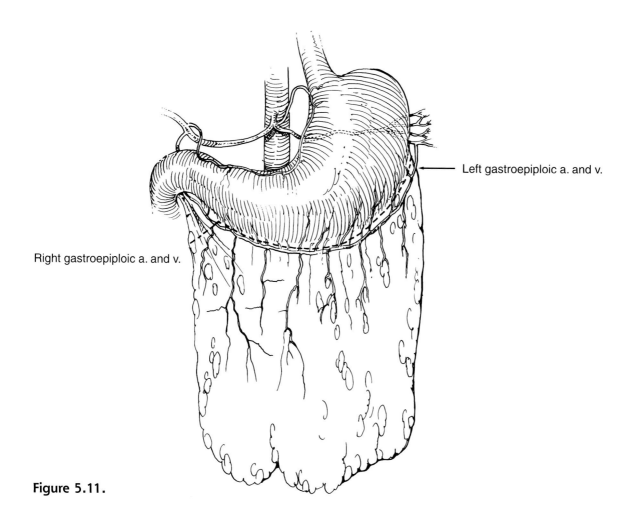

Left gastroepiploic a. and v.

Right gastroepiploic a. and v.

Figure 5.11.

Figure 5.11–5.13. The greater omentum can be used for flap coverage of the mediastinal wound based on the right or the left gastroepiploic vessels. Usually the right gastroepiploic vessels are preferred and the flap is tunneled through a central diaphragmatic incision.

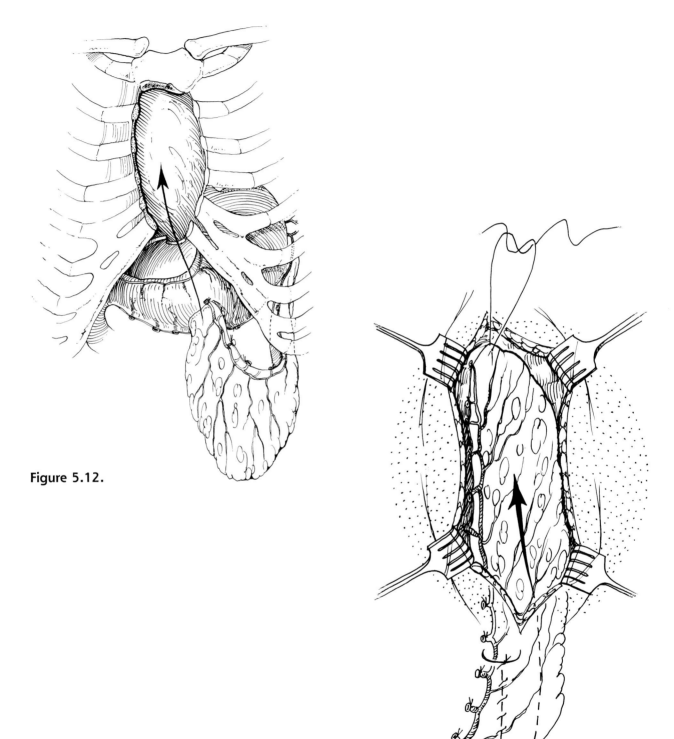

Figure 5.12.

Figure 5.13.

toralis minor muscle. Additional vessels nourish the pectoralis major, including the lateral thoracic artery to the lateral and inferior portions of the muscle, the superior thoracic artery to the clavicular portion, and the intercostal perforators from the internal mammary artery. The thoracoacromial artery first courses laterally from the midclavicle for approximately 4 cm and then turns along a line extending from the acromion to the xiphisternum.[4] This dominant artery is accompanied by venae comitantes and the lateral pectoral nerve.

Because of its vascular anatomy, the pectoralis can be classified as a Mathes–Nahai type V muscle.[5] As such, it can survive on a superolateral or thoracoacromial pedicle, or it can be based on its medial or internal mammary–intercostal perforator blood supply. This vascular arrangement makes the muscle amenable to segmental use, especially when the internal mammary perforators are preserved.

TECHNIQUE

Aggressive debridement must be performed to rid the wound of foreign bodies and contaminated and/or desiccated tissues—especially cartilage and bone—as an essential first step of wound reconstruction. All involved sternum must be removed with an adequate margin of grossly normal bone. Any costal cartilage that is exposed, contaminated, or desiccated must be removed to its bony—cartilaginous junction because of poor tolerance to desiccation or contamination. These cartilages are the most common cause of recurrent infection or drainage. The heart, great vessels, and mediastinal pleura are curetted also to remove debris and diminish the level of contamination within the wound.

If copious purulent drainage is found, or if active wound or generalized sepsis is present, it is sometimes necessary to defer flap reconstruction at the same sitting and instead stage the needed procedures. Thus, an initial debridement is followed by a period of topical care before definitive closure is performed. It is also ideal to administer culture-directed antibiotics perioperatively.

The potential space that is formed by the debridement should be obturated with well-vascularized tissue—in this case the pectoralis major. Depending on the three-dimensional geometry of the wound and where the preponderance of "dead space" is, a variety of choices can be made regarding the use of the pectoralis major. If it is used as a thoracoacromial-based advancement flap, the tendinous insertion may be divided if greater mobility is required. If it is divided, its lateral remnant may be secured to the lateral chest wall by the method that Nahai used to simulate an anterior axillary fold.

Another option is the use of the pectoralis turnover flap. Either the advancement or the turnover flap can to a great extent be split in the direction of the muscle fibers to make separate flap components or segments, each of which may be inset in somewhat different locations. Combinations of both pectoralis advancement and turnover flaps may be employed in any given wound, as they may complement each other.

If the turnover flap is used, care must be taken, of course, to make certain that the vascular supply of the perforators through the internal mammary system has not been interrupted. This often occurs with the popular use of the internal mammary as a conduit for coronary revascularization. The internal mammary artery may also be injured in the debridement. If the injury is a focal one, it is still often possible to utilize a segment of the muscle based on collateral flow via the intercostal vessels. Thus, it is critical for the reconstructive surgeon to either perform or closely observe the debridement and be aware of the details of other prior interventions to be fully aware of the vascular anatomy.

The pectoral sternocostal origins are identified and their dissection initiated. The areolar space deep to the subpectoral muscle is entered. This loose areolar space is then developed with digital dissection once the dissection of the origins has been completed with the electrocautery. If a pectoralis muscle flap and not a musculocutaneous flap is to be used to obturate the wound, the superficial pectoralis is first bared by dissecting cutaneous flaps from its surface with a combination of blunt, sharp, and cautery dissection.

Next, the vascular pedicle is clearly identified with a lighted retractor in a distinctive, small, infraclavicular, submuscular fat pad at the site described above in Anatomy. The remainder of the dissection of the flap is performed, dividing the humeral insertion and/or the clavicular attachments as needed to deliver the tissue to the central chest wound. If the muscle can be transposed or advanced adequately without complete skeletonization of the pedicle, a cuff of muscle at the pedicle will help protect it from undue traction. Again, depending on the needs of the wound, the pectoralis muscle fibers may be partially divided in their direction to provide segmental muscle flaps for delivery to various segments of the wound.

If a pectoralis turnover flap is to be utilized, the humeral insertion is divided as well. It is helpful either to utilize a lighted retractor or suction and electrocautery extender or to perform an axillary counter-incision to adequately visualize this area. To allow the flap to be turned over, the dominant thoracoacromial pedicle is doubly ligated and divided and the entire clavicular origin of the muscle incised as well. This allows for reflection of the muscle about its medial axis. All the fibers at the humeral end of the muscle are tethered together when medial reflection of a turnover flap is performed. Therefore, in this form the muscle is most reliably delivered to the central portion of the wound. If, however, it is desired to deliver additional bulk to more inferior or superior locations, the flap can be split along the direction of its fibers, as described above, to provide segmental turnover flaps and more evenly distribute the muscle to other territories in the wound.

If rectus abdominis flaps are required as well, these are elevated on the internal mammary–superior epigastric axis. The flaps are then inset to optimally utilize and distribute their tissue within the wound, best filling the resectional defect that has been created. Several different arrangements or possible patterns of inset can be simulated with the tissue to best determine the ideal use and situation of the muscles. These muscles are then secured to each other and to remnants of periosteum or perichondrium with absorbable sutures.

Careful attention must be paid to hemostasis in the flap donor site especially, because dramatic potential spaces with large raw surfaces are created by flap elevation. Multiple suction catheters are then placed via separate stab wounds to drain the flap donor sites as well as the central mediastinal recipient site.

Meticulous cutaneous closure is then performed with a layer of buried absorbable dermal sutures and a layer of running monofilament nonabsorbable sutures. The air- and watertight nature of the closure should be confirmed to prevent contamination of the large contiguous bipectoral–mediastinal space. This closure is truly critical when pectoral cutaneous flaps are secured over separate pectoralis muscle flaps, in which case the immense potential space is much closer to the surface.

When stable, the patient can be extubated. Careful attention must be paid to the suction catheters so as to prevent the complication of postoperative fluid collection. The patient should be mobilized as early as possible after an initial period of observations. If the humeral insertions of the pectoralis muscles were not divided, arm abduction is restricted in the early postoperative course to minimize tension on the muscle closure.

PITFALLS

The pectoralis is generally considered a reliable and useful flap. Failure to identify the vascular pedicle will, of course, result in flap failure. This pedicle is usually apparent on the undersurface of the muscle and is best seen with the lighted retractor or suction tip. It is found to be within a characteristic, unique, yellowish fat pad. Injury to the pedicle can most easily occur as the humeral insertion is being divided and dissection transition is being made to division of clavicular fibers. Over-skeletonization of the pedicle with traction can also result in embarrassment of the flap circulation.

In the great majority of cases, even wide cutaneous dehiscences can be closed with overlying pectoral cutaneous advancement flaps. In patients with severe diabetes or untreated nutritional compromise, and *especially* in those with weighty breasts, the central cutaneous incision can be prone to disruption. When breast weight is a problem, use of a brassiere immediately postoperatively can help support the wound. The problem can also be considered a somewhat relative contraindication to the use of pectoralis flaps in severe macromastia. In cases such as these, use of the rectus abdominis or the greater omentum should be considered. In the obese, severely diabetic patient, isolated instances of partial or total breast necrosis can occur with macromastia.

DISCUSSION

Sternal wounds, once a dreaded complication of cardiac surgery, are now eminently reconstructible with modern flap techniques. With attention to surgical principles of aggressive preoperative preparation, adequate debridement, and obturation and closure of the defect with well-vascularized tissues, this goal is accomplished with a minimum of morbidity.

Although the pectoralis muscle has been established as the workhorse of anterior chest wall reconstruction, its use is not indicated in *all* central anterior thoracic settings. Use of the rectus abdominis is indicated, for example, when tissue is needed in the epigastric region or a central, vertically oriented, relatively narrow mediastinal wound. At times, one or both rectus abdominis muscles alone will suffice to address such wounds, avoiding the need to incur the potential space of a pectoral dissection. Avoidance of the pectoral dissection is especially helpful in cases of macromastia or in the presence of other such factors.

The greater omentum[6] is a valuable flap in similar cases, including sternal wounds in patients with macromastia. Furthermore, the omentum is excellent in salvage cases or in cases in which prior interventions have violated other flap donor sites.

The latissimus dorsi muscle can be used for anterior mediastinal reconstruction, but requires extensive mobilization, skeletonization, and intraoperative turning of the patient. The aforementioned flaps are clearly preferred in most cases.

Roundtable Discussion

Dr. Stahl

We have evolved clear-cut indications for closure of mediastinal wounds since the late 1970s. The pectoralis has been established as the standard flap of anterior chest wall and mediastinal reconstruction. It is very versatile in terms of being used as an advancement or a turnover flap or being able to be split to deliver various parts of the muscle to specific locations in the wound.

One thing that is often neglected in talking about the treatment of any wound is the thoroughness with which the debridement must be pursued. No muscle flap can cure an established osteomyelitis without proper resection of the wound itself. The resection must include the sternum and/or involved costal cartilages. We have to be definitive and proceed beyond the tissues that are grossly involved in the disease process, especially in terms of costal cartilage resection. It is well known that the cartilages tolerate infection or desiccation very poorly. It is important to adequately debride these well away from the wound, if not to the bony–cartilaginous junctions of the ribs. Not only does this help eradicate abnormal areas, but if there is a wound separation postoperatively, the remoteness of these debridement margins will help guarantee that secondary healing of these small residual open wounds will proceed without difficulty.

Even though the pectoralis is well established as our workhorse, we would be remiss in not mentioning some of the other units that provide us with critical areas of coverage that the pectoralis may not be able to address. This is especially true of the lower third of the wound or long, vertical, narrow wounds, where rectus abdominis is invaluable. Greater omentum and, to a lesser extent, latissimus are units that can also be used. We also have to take care in elevating these flaps to make certain, of course, that the vascular supply is adequate. In these days when the internal mammary artery is well established as a conduit of choice for coronary revascularization, we have to be sure that rectus abdominis or pectoralis flaps are well nourished and that this issue is addressed in terms of adequate collateral flow and so on, so that we don't end up with a useless flap at the end of the case. Finally, one last point that I would like to make is that the reconstructive surgeon has to witness or participate in the debridement to ascertain the status of the internal mammary artery.

Dr. Elliott

The pectoralis is versatile, especially when it is split—used as a turnover flap or based on the thoracoacromial pedicle, as you described. But there are large planes of dissection opened up for a bilateral pectoralis coverage and that concerns me in terms of subsequent hematoma, seroma, or wound infection. I find that use of the rectus flap avoids these problems. The flap is long and satisfies the lower third all the way up to the sternal notch without difficulty. On the other hand, although I know it can be accomplished if the internal mammary on that side has been taken, I don't think it is as reliable in a very sick patient. In that case, I go to the omentum as my second choice after the rectus. The pectoralis is now my third choice in most large wounds, but in a small, limited sternal wound in the upper half to one-third I would still use the pectoralis.

It should be mentioned that the omentum can be developed even after laparotomy, especially gynecologic laparotomies. I don't debride the entire sternum in almost any case, but I agree that if the cartilages are exposed from previous partial or complete sternectomies, they need to be debrided. Drainage is very important both above and below the flap, but below the flap I would use a thin Jackson–Pratt-type drain to obliterate the dead space and I think that's an opportunity for failure of your operation.

Dr. Toth

I don't understand your concern about broad tissue planes and concerns for infection in raising bilateral pectoral flaps; you have a low threshold to go to a separate body cavity. I have found that the pectoralis major, even in lower-third sternal defects, assuming one internal mammary is open, is all that one needs. It is a rare situation in my experience to ever need to go beyond the pectoral muscles for sternal closure. For the lower third of the sternum it is a misconception that you cannot get good pectoralis major to that location. It has to be used as a turnover flap with division of the upper two sternocostal perforators. The dissection must also extend to the insertion of the humerus; as it is turned over, the flap will extend to the lower third of the sternum. Your point is well taken with regard to going to the omentum. Since patency rates with internal mammary revascularization are better than with saphenous vein interposition grafting, we run into this situation commonly when both internal mammaries have been taken. In this instance, the rectus abdominis is a less reliable choice for lower third, the pectoralis may not be a choice, and certainly omentum then moves to the top of your list.

Dr. Moses

I think that in my hands the rectus abdominis is the workhorse for a sternal wound infection. The only downside to it is an additional skin scar on the abdomen, which, considering the magnitude of the problem, is not much of a loss. I feel that it is a better fit to the contour of the wound and that there is a significant functional loss in the sacrifice of one or both pectoralis muscles in terms of upper extremity function that is not encountered when the rectus abdominis muscle is sacrificed.

Dr. Grotting

With respect to timing, the wounds that break down and begin to drain the first 7 days after a bypass, or an emergency sternotomy, are in general a different group. These are patients who have acute infection where the wound is not stable. In these patients we have had better success, especially if there has been any fresh pus involved, in doing one or more initial debridements, and then going ahead with definitive closure. P.G. Arnold has made the case that this is not a debridement procedure, but a resection. In their very large series of cases, their failures almost all occurred in patients who had had subtotal debridements of the wound and had not had resection. In patients who had total sternal resection and resection of the costal cartilages, the rate of success was virtually 100%—this is the key to this procedure.

By the advancement of pectoralis musculocutaneous units, that is, dissecting under the pectoralis muscle, advancing muscle and the skin as a unit—not dividing the humeral insertion, not turning the flap over—but simply bringing the muscle and skin together, these can be handled simply. It is not necessary to close all the dead space in this type of wound. It is unique in that regard.

We have had trouble with the rectus. We started out thinking that the rectus would be an ideal solution for this; but in patients who are debilitated, obese, or diabetic, there can be substantial donor site problems with the use of the rectus and so we have restricted the use of the rectus to very, very specific indications. The omentum, likewise, needs to be brought through either the anterior fascia or the diaphragm, and this is a problematic area, particularly in a patient who is ventilator dependent, and one can experience dehiscences and eviscerations through that particular tunnel, particularly when the omentum has just been skin grafted.

Dr. Stahl

With regard to this dead-space issue, debridement actually helps reduce the dead space in terms of the geometry of the wound. It makes a more lateral shelf across which any kind of flap must be passed, and this is another matter with which debridement can help—not just to rid the wound of contamination but to help flaps be inset with greater ease and effectiveness. Some of the pitfalls of the use of the pectoralis lie with some of these high-risk patients, such as those mentioned in this chapter—especially those with large, heavy, pendulous breasts in whom we have to worry about the donor sites.

REFERENCES

1. Bryant LB, Spencer FC, Trinkle JK. Treatment of median sternotomy infection by mediastinal irrigation with an antibiotic solution. Ann Surg 1969;169:914.

2. Shumacker HB, Mandelbaum I. Continuous antibiotic irrigation in the treatment of infection. Arch Surg 1963;83:384.

3. Jurkiewicz MJ, Krizek TJ, Mathes S, Ariyan S. Infected median sternotomy wound: Successful treatment by muscle flaps. Ann Surg 1980;191:738.

4. Ariyan S. The pectoralis major myocutaneous flap: A versatile flap for reconstruction in the head and neck, Plast Reconstr Surg 1979;63:73.

5. Mathes S, Nahai F. Clinical atlas of muscle and musculocutaneous flaps. St. Louis: C.V. Mosby, 1979:318–328.

6. Arnold PG, Irons GB. The greater omentum: Extension in transposition and free transfer. Plast Reconstr Surg 1981;67:169.

6

CLOSURE OF INTRATHORACIC WOUNDS

JAMES H. FRENCH, JR.

THE PROBLEM

The patient is an adult man with respiratory failure who developed a distal tracheal perforation. Bedside bronchoscopy confirmed the presence of a 4-cm perforation of the posterior membranous trachea down to the level of the tracheal bifurcation. Subsequent esophagoscopy was performed and was interpreted as normal to 25 cm from the incisors. The problem is an isolated distal tracheal tear that serves as a source of contamination for the adjacent tissues and represents a life-threatening situation in this patient.

INTRODUCTION

Wounds that are located in the intrathoracic space are generally complex and life-threatening. The location of or access to the wound and the inevitable sequelae or consequences of inadequate management make such wounds complex by definition. Coverage of wounds of the intrathoracic space can be obtained by using tissues from inside or outside the pleural cavity.[1-5] Flaps fashioned from pleura have long been used to cover small intrathoracic wounds. In such cases the pleura is usually thickened as a result of local inflammatory reaction and provides little more than superficial covering of the wound in question. Pleural flaps do not have the advantages that accompany muscle flaps, i.e., increased vascularity, reliability, and adequate bulk.

The goal in the management of the case illustrated is to provide a well-vascularized repair of the posterior tracheal wound, and to do so in such a way as to prevent further contamination by the trachea and thus to minimize surgical morbidity.

The serratus anterior muscle was selected as the vascularized tissue of choice. Its proven reliability and specific characteristics make it a logical choice in this particular case.

ANATOMY

The serratus anterior muscle is a flat muscle that functions as a stabilizer for the scapula. It originates from the outer surface of the upper eight or nine ribs and inserts along the inferior and medial border of the scapula.[6] The nerve supply is via the long thoracic nerve that arises from C-5, C-6, and C-7. It courses inferiorly along the serratus fascia, joining the serratus branch of the thoracodorsal artery at about the level of the sixth slip.[7] The muscle has a dual blood supply. The lateral thoracic artery, which is the second branch of the axillary artery, enters the lateral surface of the muscle and supplies the upper four or five slips. The second vessel that serves as a blood supply for the muscle is the thoracodorsal artery. This artery enters the posterolateral aspect of the muscle and supplies the lower three slips (Figure 6.1).[6,7]

Releasing the origin and insertion gives the muscle an arc of rotation that will allow the it to reach most ipsilateral intrathoracic, anterior chest, and shoulder areas. It also can be used as a free tissue transfer for coverage or function. As long as its upper portion is kept intact, the use of the lower

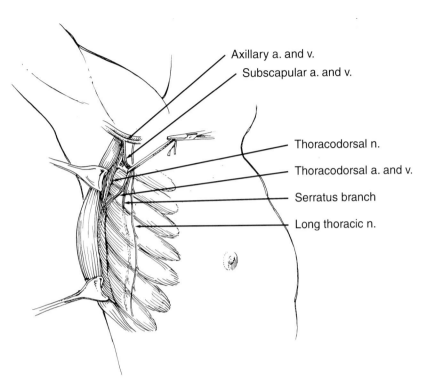

Figure 6.1. Anatomy, innervation, and blood supply of serratus anterior muscle.

slips has little effect on function.[7] Loss of function of the muscle results in a winged scapula.

Technique

The patient is placed in a lateral decubitus position, and the incision to be used depends on the patient's postoperative status, that is, whether or not he or she has had a previous thoracotomy. If a previous lateral thoracotomy has been performed, then the old incision can be used to gain access to the serratus anterior muscle. If the patient has not had a thoracotomy, then a standard thoracotomy incision can be performed in such a way as to preserve the latissimus dorsi muscle. That would allow the latissimus muscle to be a secondary choice if the serratus anterior muscle cannot be used. In those cases in which the serratus anterior muscle is used as a free-tissue transfer, such as a contralateral wound, the incision is planned in a vertical direction approximately 4 cm anterior to the posterior axillary fold.[7] However, most cases involve situations in which the muscle is needed for ipsilateral wound coverage and the patient has had a lateral thoracotomy or a lateral thoracotomy is planned. Therefore, the old incision is used. The divided latissimus dorsi muscle is identified and the proximal segment is easily separated from the underlying serratus anterior muscle. It is reflected superiorly and the latissimus dorsi branch of the thoracodorsal artery is identified. The vessel is traced proximally and the branch of the serratus anterior muscle is located. The thoracodorsal branch is part of the dual blood supply to the muscle. It supplies the lower portion, whereas the lateral thoracic artery supplies the upper part. The muscle is elevated off the chest wall along its anterior and inferior attachments (Figure 6.2). The entire dissection of this muscle flap is best done with the cautery except for the dissection around the vascular pedicle.

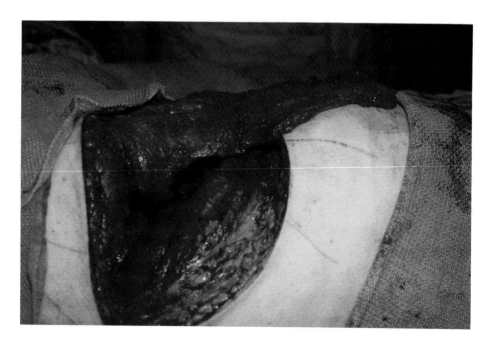

Figure 6.2. Serratus anterior muscle draped over thoracotomy prior to insertion.

The posterolateral attachments that involve the medial and inferior aspect of the scapula are severed. In addition, the serratus anterior and latissimus dorsi muscles interdigitate inferiorly, and this area is also divided with the cautery. As is the case in many posterolateral thoracotomies, a midlevel rib (such as the fifth rib) is removed for purposes of exposure. A more proximal window is needed for the serratus anterior muscle and, therefore, a segment of the second rib can be removed, providing access for the muscle (Figure 6.3). An alternative approach is an incision in the second intercostal space. In a patient with an unusually thick serratus anterior muscle or narrow intercostal space, introducing the muscle into the pleural space via an intercostal window instead of a partial rib excision would possibly create a vascular compromise of the flap. If there is any question about the size of the window, part of the rib should be removed. By allowing the muscle to enter at this point, most areas of the pleural space can be reached. The muscle is then used to reinforce and/or cover the

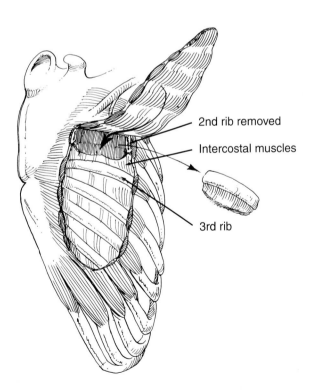

2nd rib removed

Intercostal muscles

3rd rib

Figure 6.3. Serratus anterior flap elevated, second rib removed.

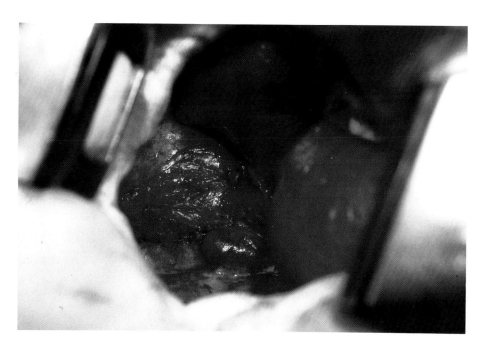

Figure 6.4. Serratus anterior muscle sewn in place.

wounds (Figure 6.4). Nonabsorbable suture, such as Prolene, is used to hold the muscle in place. In repair of the trachea or bronchial tree, the repair is tested with a positive ventilatory pressure. The pleural space is then copiously irrigated with antibiotic solution and closed in routine layered fashion over two pleural drainage tubes (Figures 6.5 and 6.6).

DISCUSSION

The principles of management of intrathoracic wounds are no different than those of wounds in other parts of the body. Experimentally, muscle flaps have been used successfully in pigs to repair aortic defects.[8] In addition, intercostal muscle flaps have been used for repair of induced cardiac defects in dogs.[9] In clinical situations, tracheal, esophageal, and bronchopleural fistulas, as well as active or impending vascular problems, have been managed with muscular tissue.[1-5] Also, wounds with exposed cardiac

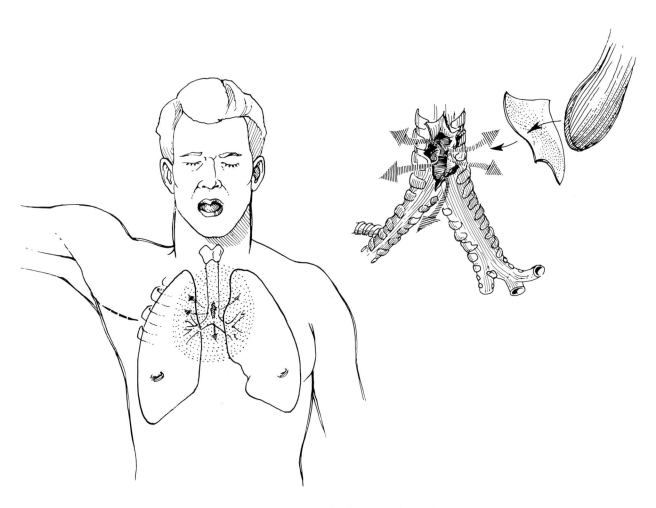

Figure 6.5.   Demonstration of injury and coverage with pleura and muscle flap.

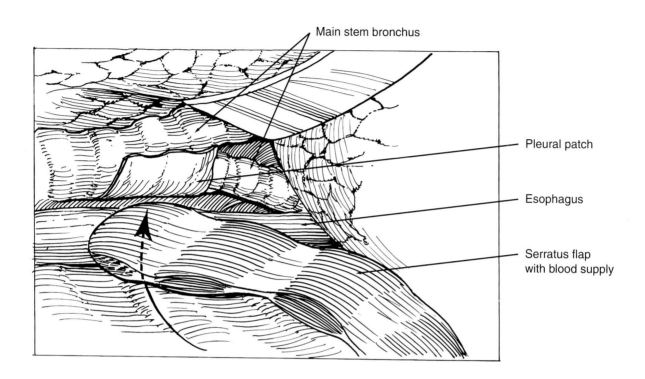

Main stem bronchus

Pleural patch

Esophagus

Serratus flap with blood supply

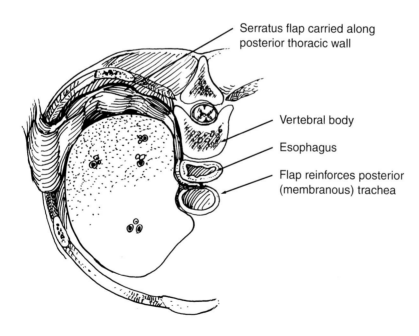

Serratus flap carried along posterior thoracic wall

Vertebral body

Esophagus

Flap reinforces posterior (membranous) trachea

Figure 6.6. Demonstration of muscle placement.

prostheses have been successfully closed with the help of muscle coverage.[10]

Conceptually, muscle flaps that are used for external thoracic wound coverage should be able to be utilized with corresponding intrathoracic wounds. Muscles that have been used for such procedures include the pectoralis major, latissimus dorsi, serratus anterior, rectus abdominis, and intercostal muscles.[1-5] As in any wound management, coverage with a free tissue transfer is a possibility but rarely need be a consideration in this particular case.

There are several practical reasons the serratus anterior muscle is desirable for management of such intrathoracic problems. It is a broad, thin muscle that is easily raised and transposed into the pleural space. The muscle has a dual blood supply and potentially a very long pedicle if the flap is raised in the thoracodorsal vessel. If need be, the function of the muscle can be preserved by harvesting only the inferior slips of the muscle. In addition, it is often spared during a lateral thoracotomy where the latissimus dorsi muscle is often divided.

A restrictive pulmonary problem is the theoretical consideration when planning intrathoracic coverage of the serratus muscle flap. However, this has not been experienced in the clinical setting. Again, the size of the serratus anterior muscle makes it ideal for the pleural space. In addition, many of the patients in whom the flap was indicated have had partial or total pulmonary resection, which provides room for the flap.

Inadequate length should not be a problem with the serratus anterior muscle. If need be, the pedicle can be lengthened by having a flap based only on a thoracodorsal branch. This maneuver should allow the muscle to reach the potential problems along the medial aspect of the pleural space.

Winged scapula is an unfortunate sequela to this operation. However, most of the cases in which the serratus anterior flap is needed are life-threatening, and therefore, the winged scapula can be considered a fair compromise. The winged scapula can be avoided if only the inferior three slips are used and proximal innervation is maintained.

Summary

In summary, the serratus anterior muscle is an excellent choice for muscle coverage of intrathoracic wounds. Its size, shape, and pedicle allow the muscle access to the problem areas of the pleural space. In addition, its accessibility during routine lateral thoracotomy and its reliability support its use as the muscle of choice for intrathoracic wound management. The flap is easily raised and transposed to the intrathoracic area of concern. Winged scapula is the most profound side effect and should be considered in the preoperative planning of the intrathoracic wound management. Raising the flap is relatively easy using the cautery throughout dissection, except for the dissection around the pedicles. Exposure is not a problem using standard intrathoracic restriction. Testing repair of the trachea or a portion of the bronchial tree with positive ventilatory pressure helps confirm the reliability of the repair. And finally, using pleural flaps as initial cover provides an extra layer for the repair, which should not be considered the heart of the repair.

Roundtable Discussion

Dr. French

This serratus anterior flap was selected in this particular case because of the size of the flap. It's a thin muscle that can be used in the wound that is in an intrathoracic space. In this case, the wound is located in the medial aspect of the intrathoracic space and it was easily elevated and transposed into this space. Other flaps were considered in this particular case. The latissimus muscle had been divided and so was not an option.

Dr. Elliott

I agree that the serratus is wonderful because of its proximity to what you're trying to cover. In my mind there are two settings for coverage of intrathoracic problems. One is an acute problem such as a tracheal blowout or an acute bronchial pleural fistula. The other is the empyema cavity that develops a bronchopleural fistula where you've got both the fistula itself and a cavity, or something of that sort, in which there's a large hole in the chest. The serratus is much larger than you think and not usually divided by the thoracotomy incision. You can bring it in up high and it works nicely. I've also used the omentum tunneled up either through the diaphragm or subcutaneously to cover a bronchopleural fistula, and that works very nicely when the serratus may not be enough because of the high thoracotomy incision. In the delayed situation or the chronic situation in which you have an empyema cavity associated with it, the results at the Mayo Clinic with regard to simply filling the cavity with antibiotic solution and closing the wound do seem to work in a large majority of cases. In some of those cases you do want to fill and obliterate the space, and I've used the transverse rectus abdominis myocutaneous (TRAM) flap along with the serratus flap—the serratus first to close the fistula and follow with the TRAM flap to obturate the cavity.

Dr. Stahl

We usually don't have a choice about whether or not that latissimus has been divided by the thoracic surgeon. In developing a close relationship with the thoracic surgeons, though, we can influence the thoracic surgeon to do latissimus-sparing thoracotomies. Secondly, I think that, depending on the location of the wound, we sometimes sell our latissimus remnant short. In the posterolateral thoracotomies it just looks as if that whole latissimus is going to be totally useless, but I think it's good to use if a supplement to the serratus is needed. Another point is that rib resection is helpful for exposure, to allow for passage of the flap into the cavity and then finally, in terms of unroofing the cavity adequately to allow for full obturation of the wound.

DR. ZUBOWICZ

I agree emphatically with what Dr. Stahl just said. Secondly the more common problem in my practice is the patient who has dead space, generally from empyema with an air leak, and I find that transfer of remnants of the latissimus and serratus usually does well in obliterating dead space. My question is, How do you manage the suction catheter between the chest wall and these muscle flaps? It generates negative pressure, and in the patient with an air leak, is that not going to contribute to the muscle pulling away and exacerbating the problem? What I've done is to pack that dead space, allow the muscles to stick to the hilum and the lung, and then come back and close that secondarily. Is that an agreed-upon method of treatment?

DR. FRENCH

I haven't done that procedure, but it certainly makes sense. In the cases with which I've been involved, the suction catheters have not created a problem, and the muscle has remained against the fistula or the wound. I've never packed these wounds to obliterate the dead space. Usually I've done it with either the muscle flaps or deepithelialized tissue, as Dr. Elliott mentioned.

DR. TOTH

I agree with your choice of flap for a solution here, and I think in general the point needs to be made that most of these patients are extremely sick because of the nature of their disease. Thus, whenever possible, using tissue that is in and around the wound that you have created to address the problem is much better than going to distant sites, and taking abdominal or intraabdominal tissue adds morbidity in a compromised patient. I would first use the latissimus remnant or the serratus with overlying deepithelialized tissue if necessary before looking elsewhere.

DR. FRENCH

I would like to ask the group if anyone has used an intercostal flap before?

DR. STAHL

Actually, Dr. French, I was going to add that when Dr. Zubowicz talked about packing the wound and difficulties with air leak and securing the muscle flap into the recipient bed. Pairolero and Arnold have advocated packing the wound as Dr. Zubowicz suggested. The intercostal flaps have helped me secure these tissues, the latissimus remnant or serratus, with some pressure in a more formal controllable manner. They can thus really be used to help buttress or closure. So I would agree with that, and I'm glad you brought it up.

DR. STAHL

As I understood it, you used the pleural flap as a partition and for mechanical purposes, but relied on the muscle flaps as the vascularized reconstruction.

DR. FRENCH

That's correct.

DR. STAHL

Dr. French, we always worry about the winged scapular donor deformity, and you very properly mentioned it in your chapter. In your practice, have you seen this as a real problem or complaint?

DR. FRENCH

The people that we have used the flap on have been very sick patients. This was a life-saving measure and that has not been a complaint. But I think many times it's more the concern of the surgeon than it is of the patient for this particular problem.

DR. STAHL

That would be my impression also, in that I always talk to the patient about it and worry about it myself. But I haven't really seen it as a problem either. I wonder if we worry about it too much in these settings.

DR. McKINNON

What did you feel were your alternatives in this situation and those that approximate this one?

DR. FRENCH

I think there are several alternatives. The alternatives would be the latissimus remnant, the rectus abdominis, and perhaps the intercostal muscles.

DR. MCKINNON

Do you do an arteriogram to make sure that the blood supply to the latissimus is intact in a secondary case?

DR. FRENCH

No, I suppose you could do that, but I think you should be able to tell by the incision or by the scar if they've crossed the latissimus.

DR. STAHL

One other flap that should be on the list, depending on the wound location, is the pectoralis major. It can be dropped through a window, getting a lot of mileage out of that in certain cases. So that's just one other thing to add. It's commonly not described that much for lateral thoracic wounds. It is more commonly helpful in the mediastinitis setting, but it can be of help in some situations.

REFERENCES

1. Demos NJ, Timmes JJ. Myoplasty for closure of tracheal bronchial fistula. Ann Thorac Surg 1973;15:88.

2. Hankins JR, Miller JE, McLaughlin JS. The use of chest wall muscle flaps to close bronchopleural fistulas: Experience with 21 patients. Ann Thorac Surg 1978;25:491.

3. Pairolero PC, Arnold PG. Bronchopleural fistula: Treatment by transposition of pectoralis major muscle. J Thorac Cardiovasc Surg 1983;86:809.

4. Pairolero PC, Arnold PG, Piehler JM. Intrathoracic transposition of extrathoracic skeletal muscle. J Thorac Cardiovasc Surg 1983;86:809.

5. Arnold PG, Pairolero PC, Waldorf JC. The serratus anterior muscle: Intrathoracic and extrathoracic utilization. Plast Reconstr Surg 1984;73:240.

6. Arnold PG, Pairolero PC. Intrathoracic muscle flaps: A ten-year experience in the management of life-threatening infections. Plast Reconstr Surg 1989; 92.

7. Mathes SJ, Nahai F. Clinical atlas of muscle and musculocutaneous flaps. St. Louis: C.V. Mosby Co., 1979:337–345.

8. Grotting J. Microvascular Transfer of the Serratus Anterior Muscle. In: Grabb's Encyclopedia of Flaps: 608–612.

9. Horneffer PJ, French JH, Hutchins GM, Gardner TJ. The use of muscle flaps in the repair of aortic defects. J Thorac Cardiovasc Surg 1985;90:361–366.

10. Papp C, Parker P, Boeheim C, McGraw JB. Experimental use of intercostal muscle flaps for repair of induced cardiac defects. Submitted for publication.

11. French J. Coverage of exposed cardiac prostheses. Presentation at Northeastern Society of Plastic Surgeons, Philadelphia, 1984.

4

DECISION MAKING
IN
UPPER EXTREMITY
RECONSTRUCTION

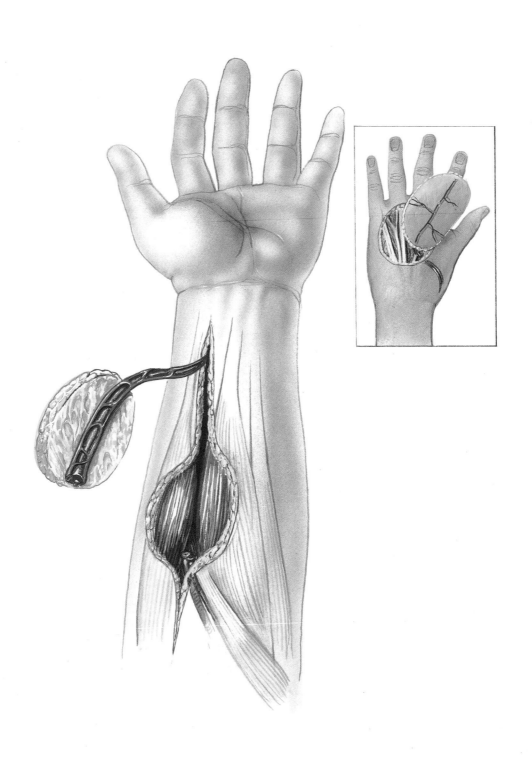

Forearm Coverage with Free Latissimus Muscle Flap and Skin Graft

James C. Grotting and Carl C. Askren

The Problem

The patient was a 27-year-old man who was involved in a motorcycle accident that resulted in a posterior dislocation at the elbow and loss of pulsatile flow in the radial and ulnar vessels. Additionally, he had impaired neurologic function in the median and radial nerve distributions. There was extensive swelling of the proximal forearm and antecubital fossa (Figure 7.1a,b). Urgent exploration was undertaken to evaluate and repair the neurovascular structures.

At surgery, a fasciotomy-type incision was made extending medially over the upper arm, transversely across the antecubital fossa, and down the flexor surface to within 6 cm of the wrist flexion crease. A large hematoma was found in the deep tissues of the forearm. There was disruption of the brachial artery just proximal to the bifurcation. Deep veins of the forearm were also disrupted. The major nerves were found to be contused but intact. In addition, the origin of the flexor musculator had been disrupted. The brachial artery reconstruction was carried out with a saphenous vein graft by the vascular surgery service. Twenty-four hours postoperatively the pulses in the hand disappeared.

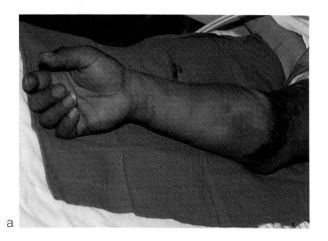
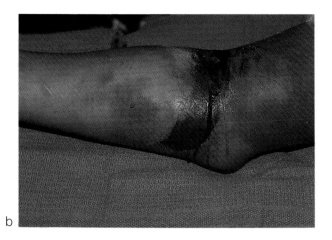

a

b

Figure 7.1.(a,b).   Blunt injury to elbow resulting in brachial artery avulsion and devascularization of forearm and hand. Note the devitalized skin over the antecubital fossa.

INTRODUCTION

Injuries of the forearm, as in the hand, may range from simple skin and subcutaneous tissue avulsions to more complex injuries that threaten upper extremity amputation. This chapter focuses on a severe devascularizing injury of the upper extremity and the selection of a unique flap for coverage.

The patient was urgently returned to the operating room where exploration of the wound revealed a thrombosed vein graft. Overlying nonviable skin was debrided (Figure 7.2). A latissimus dorsi muscle with an intact subscapular artery and circumflex scapular side branch was harvested from the contralateral side (Figure 7.3a,b). Microvascular anastomoses were carried out utilizing the subscapular and circumflex scapular vessels interposed between the brachial artery and radial–ulnar bifurcation as a flow-through flap (Figure 7.4). The perfused latissimus provided the necessary soft tissue coverage (Figure 7.5). The muscle was covered with a meshed split-thickness skin graft (Figure 7.6).

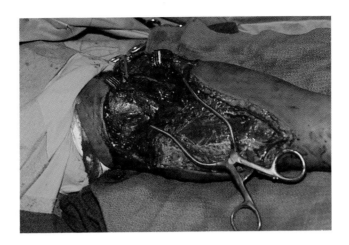

Figure 7.2. Following debridement of nonviable soft tissue and the thrombosed vein graft, the proximal and distal arterial segments are isolated.

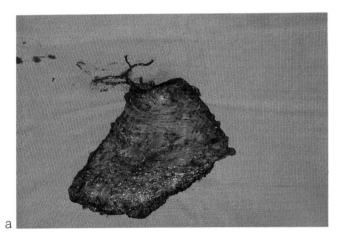

a

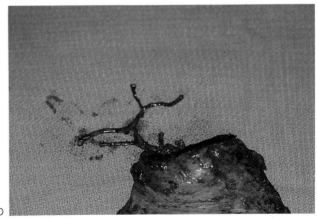

b

Figure 7.3.(a,b). The latissimus muscle arterial pedicle with a segment of the circumflex scapular artery for use as a flow-through graft.

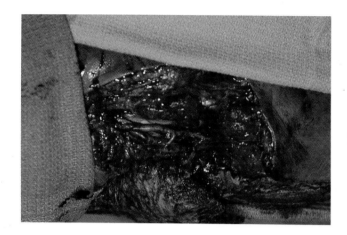

Figure 7.4. Intraoperative view illustrating the arterial reconstruction of the brachial artery using the vascular pedicle to the latissimus dorsi as a flow-through arterial graft. The latissimus muscle is well perfused.

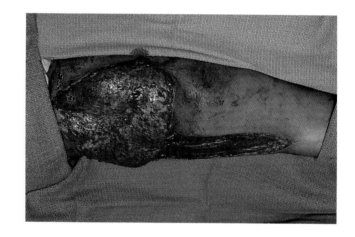

Figure 7.5. Intraoperative view of wound coverage.

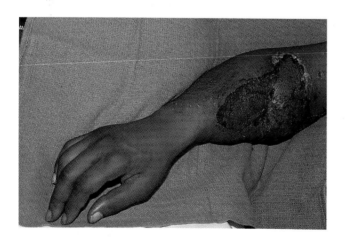

Figure 7.6. Late postoperative view of the reconstruction.

ANATOMY

The primary pedicle of the latissimus dorsi is the thoracodorsal trunk, which is about 10 cm long. The subscapular artery originates from the axillary artery. Its first branch is the circumflex scapular, and it terminates as the serratus branch and the thoracodorsal branch to the latissimus. Since its early description, the flap has been widely used and modified. By using either the circumflex scapular or the serratus branches, it may be used as a flow-through arterial graft for vascular as well as soft tissue reconstruction.

TECHNIQUE

Some traumatic injuries may result in disruption of the arterial inflow to the arm. Although a reversed saphenous vein graft could be used to repair a segmental loss of the brachial artery, the reconstructed vessel and its anastomoses must have satisfactory soft tissue coverage. When accompanied by soft tissue loss, vascular injuries present a difficult reconstructive challenge. The latissimus dorsi free muscle flap and the subscapular axis provide a means of revascularizing the extremity and providing soft tissue coverage simultaneously.

A two-team approach is generally taken to prepare the recipient site and to harvest the free flap. The latissimus muscle is harvested by one team through an oblique incision along the posterior axillary line. The incision is extended into the axilla (with a "Z" as needed) for axillary exposure (Figure 7.7). Under loupe magnification, the subscapular axis is carefully dissected out so that the subscapular artery and vein, the circumflex scapular, serratus, and thoracodorsal branches are all visualized (Figure 7.8).

A second team simultaneously debrides the wound and dissects the proximal and distal segments of the disrupted brachial artery.

Once the dissections are complete, the latissimus muscle is harvested on its vascular pedicle with the arterial flow-through graft and transferred

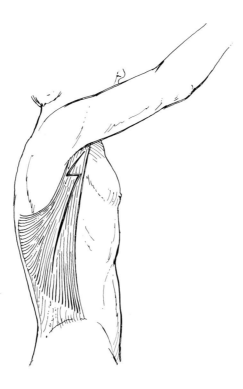

Figure 7.7. Planned incision for harvest of latissimus dorsi for free tissue transfer. "Z" extension facilitates axillary exposure.

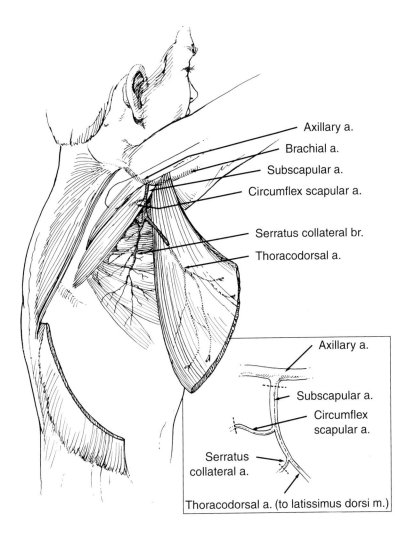

Figure 7.8. The latissimus muscle is elevated and the arterial branches are dissected to be available for the flow-through arterial graft.

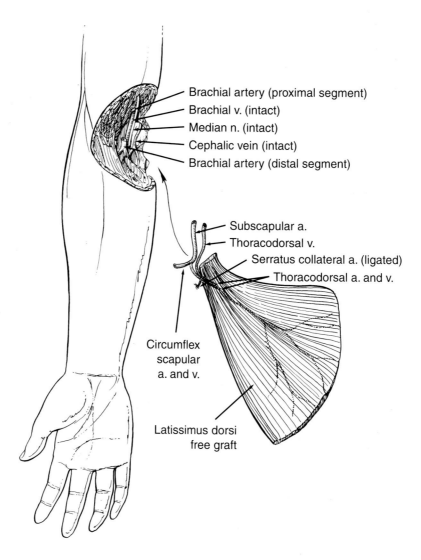

Brachial artery (proximal segment)
Brachial v. (intact)
Median n. (intact)
Cephalic vein (intact)
Brachial artery (distal segment)

Subscapular a.
Thoracodorsal v.
Serratus collateral a. (ligated)
Thoracodorsal a. and v.

Circumflex
scapular
a. and v.

Latissimus dorsi
free graft

Figure 7.9. View of flow-through arterial graft concept.

to the primary defect (Figure 7.9). The proximal microvascular anastomosis is carried out between the brachial artery and the subscapular artery. Small differences in caliber are compensated for by dilating the smaller of the two vessels (Figure 7.10). The subscapular vein can be anastomosed with a tributary of the brachial vein. Flow can then be directed into the flap, perfusing it, while the distal anastomosis is carried out between the circumflex scapular artery and the distal stump of the brachial or ulnar artery. The flow through the subscapular and circumflex scapular vessels

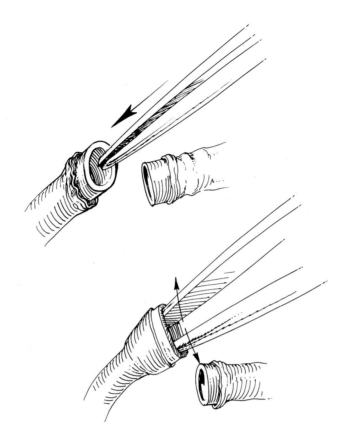

Figure 7.10. Technique of intraoperative dilation of an artery to compensate for size discrepancy.

restores continuity of blood flow to the hand, while the latissimus flap can be used to cover the soft tissue defect and the critical vascular repairs. The muscle can be tailored to fit the defect and then skin-grafted (Figure 7.11).

Discussion

The first successful free tissue transfer to the upper extremity was reported in 1974[1] and the success rate has increased over the years. Microsurgical techniques are now commonplace and much safer. Failure rates for free tissue transfer should be below 5%. The wealth of experience documented in the literature offers almost limitless choices of tissues for transplanta-

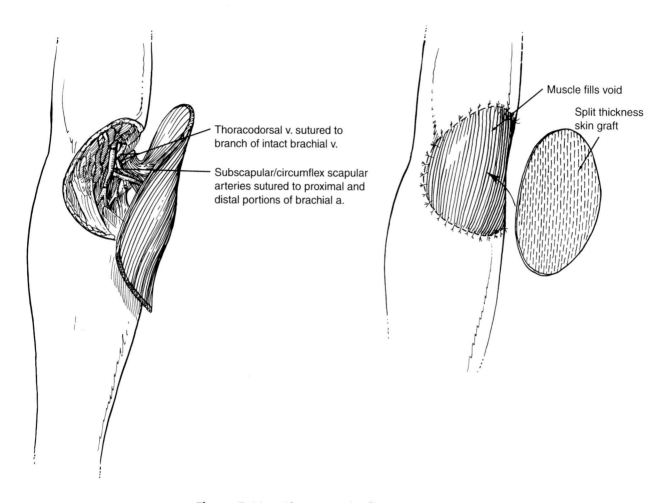

Thoracodorsal v. sutured to branch of intact brachial v.

Subscapular/circumflex scapular arteries sutured to proximal and distal portions of brachial a.

Muscle fills void

Split thickness skin graft

Figure 7.11. The composite flap is used to bridge the arterial defect with the attached latissimus muscle available for wound closure.

tion. When compared with distant flaps, free tissue transfer offers a number of advantages.[2] Free tissue transfer is a reliable technique for soft tissue coverage. Immediate revascularization is provided by the flap's own blood supply that accompanies it, in contrast to the distant flap transfer, which is dependent on the damaged recipient tissue to provide secondary revascularization. Free tissue transfer may allow not only soft tissue coverage, but bones, joints, tendons, nerves, and functional motor units may potentially be transferred simultaneously. Finally, free flaps can be precisely tailored to the needs of the defect.[3,4] The disadvantages of free flaps are that they can be time-consuming and may, like distant flaps, require revision. The free flap has thus evolved to become in many instances the procedure of choice for soft tissue coverage.

Considerations that may influence free flap choice have been outlined by Lister[5]: (1) the general health of the patient, (2) position requirements, (3) aesthetic demands of the patient, (4) the size of the wound, (5) thickness, (6) special needs of the defect, (7) the surgeon's skill, and (8) the experience of the team. The latter two are particularly important today, as proper judgment regarding the salvageability of an injured hand cannot be made without knowledge about free tissue transfer and its limitations and potential for functional restoration.

There are few absolute contraindications to flap coverage. Uncontrolled infection and dead tissue present in the wound can lead to fulminant infection if not adequately debrided. This applies to both free tissue transfer and distant flaps. Additionally, marginally vascularized recipient tissue is a contraindication to distant flaps, which are dependent on the recipient bed for vascularization.

Free tissue transfer should not be selected to cover a limb that has no potential for functional recovery. This requires a sensate hand, mobile joints, and a sufficient number of tendons and muscles. An assessment by an experienced hand surgeon must be made.

Relative contraindications include a psychiatric disturbance that may prohibit cooperation with postoperative care and rehabilitation (though in our experience, this is uncommon) or systemic disease such as end-stage diabetes, chronic obstructive pulmonary disease, or atherosclerosis. Age alone should not be a deterrent.[6]

As detailed in Chapter 6, care of the upper extremity should follow the principles of management of any trauma patient.

Postoperatively, flaps are monitored hourly by the nursing staff to assess flap warmth, turgor, color, capillary refill, and Doppler flow as detailed by the surgeon in report. The extremity is elevated and, if grafted, immobilized for an appropriate interval until graft-take is assessed as satisfactory. Mobilization is begun as early as possible without jeopardizing flaps or grafts.

Patients are placed on nasal oxygen at 2 to 4 l/min to ensure adequate oxygen delivery to the flap. Aspirin, 325 mg q.d., is begun the day following surgery. Intravenous dextran 40 in D_5W at 40 cc/h for 3 days diminishing to 20 cc/h for 2 days is optional.

Microvascular thrombosis is the major complication of free flap surgery. Salvage of a thrombosed pedicle is dependent upon early diagnosis and intervention. Continuous monitoring both intraoperatively and postoperatively on the ward is required to avoid failure of the procedure. During flap inset, a change in color may be the first indication of thrombosis. Flap skin may become pale, while muscle may change from a bright pink to a cyanotic hue.

Thrombosis of the artery may be related to arterial spasm, kinking, or inadequate inflow. Spasm may be controlled by avoiding excessive manipulation of the vessels and keeping the patient warm. Lidocain or Marcaine can be topically applied as a vasodilator. Proper alignment to avoid torsion before anastomosis and anchoring of the pedicle will prevent kinking. A sudden change in the appearance of the flap while closing may also suggest that kinking has occurred, and reexamination of the pedicle is indicated. Hypovolemia or hypotension may also result in poor flow. Decreasing the dose of inhalational agent will help to increase blood pressure to about 120 to 130 systolic, thus maintaining perfusion pressure. Venous engorgement may result in thrombosis. A vein of adequate size must be used to drain a flap. If a concomitant vein seems inadequate, a larger recipient vein should be selected and a second anastomosis should be carried out. Venous thrombosis may also result from kinking or a dressing that is too tight. Dressings should therefore be applied loosely and inspected frequently in the postoperative period.

Soft tissue coverage of larger and more complex wounds can be achieved with free tissue transfer. Unique reconstructive requirements may also be met with composite flap procedures. Early coverage, generally within the first 48 to 72 hours, is a desirable goal to achieve primary wound healing. The flow-through latissimus muscle flap can furnish arterial continuity in the acute setting of vascular compromise with soft tissue loss.

ROUNDTABLE DISCUSSION

DR. GROTTING

Microsurgery now plays a dominant role in reconstruction of the upper extremity and hand. Of course, local flaps and pedicle flaps from the groin and abdomen are available, as will be discussed in Chapter 8. We have selected as the case for discussion here a somewhat complex and rare event in which there is both devascularization and massive soft tissue loss in the area of the antecubital fossa. The reconstructive problems, then, included not only coverage of the exposed vital structures in the antecubital fossa, but also revascularization of the upper extremity following failed reverse saphenous vein bypass grafting. The concept of the case was to use an arterial graft and an attached latissimus dorsi free flap to accomplish the reconstructive goal.

DR. STAHL

I think this case is a really nice example of design, planning, and execution. It's a novel way to solve multiple problems with a single flap. I still can't help but wonder about the principles, though, of vascular reconstruction. I think the interposition of a graft, regardless of whether it's an arterial graft or a reversed venous graft, should work with application of sound vascular surgical principles. I hope that we shouldn't have to do a free flap to bail out a poor vascular result, in general, solely to achieve soft tissue coverage when it can be done more simply.

We shouldn't neglect to mention the possibility that in many cases of upper extremity tissue loss, a pedicled latissimus can reach the upper arm, and, in some cases, the antecubital region. I think this is a nice salvage, but as you mentioned, it's a rare situation that we would have the opportunity to use this method.

DR. FRENCH

The pedicled latissimus is not applicable in this case, for several reasons. First, the plan used an arterial graft. Second, the pedicled latissimus cannot be easily tunneled or inset in the upper arm to reach the elbow. Third, because of the distant pedicle, it cannot be as easily inset in the wound.

DR. MOSES

I still believe in the old-fashioned principle of replacing like with like. In this wound you have a composite of two separate problems: arterial continuity and coverage. Wouldn't it be nice if we had a piece of like tissue that involved an underlying arterial conduit and a piece of supple forearm skin? That is precisely what's missing. Exactly that unit is available in the other arm as a free forearm flap, which we all use in many circumstances. You would take as long a segment of radial artery as you wanted and have an *arterial* rather than a *venous* interposition with a well-vascularized piece of skin overlying it.

DR. GROTTING

That is a reasonable alternative, but in my mind that is simply transplanting an unacceptable defect from one arm to another. You are going to have to skin graft the donor arm, so you're trading a grafted flap on one side for a grafted donor defect on the other arm. Another thing to point out is that this wound was large, and one would have had to take virtually the whole circumference of the forearm on the opposite side to gain satisfactory coverage.

I think that the reason that arterial grafts were not so commonly used in the past is simply that arterial grafts are less available in the body and more difficult to dissect than the readily available saphenous vein graft. Also they are less expendable in the body than veins. I think this situation in which one has the opportunity to solve both problems with three anastomoses—two arterial and one venous—is better and safer than having to do four anastomoses, that is, a reversed interposition vein graft and then doing a free flap transfer. The pedicled latissimus would not have reached the distal wound margin in this particular defect.

DR. ELLIOTT

I think that replacing like with like is something we should continue to strive for, though muscle coverage of the cutaneous full-thickness problem has proved to be quite successful. In that light, a scapular flap from the opposite side using the thoracodorsal pass-through (as opposed to the circumflex scapualr pass-through) would have restored the arterial continuity *and* used skin coverage. I do agree that the size of the defect makes the scapula donor site less attractive as it gets larger. The tension on the closure would create a scar that may be more significant than a latissimus scar.

In devascularizing injuries of the proximal forearm, we have seen necrosis of the underlying flexor muscles associated with that loss of blood supply. In some of the more severe cases, we have found the extremity to be essentially unsalvageable when the flexor muscles are devascularized and necrotic. Despite the fact that arterial flow was reestablished to the hand, it can bypass all proximal flow to the muscles. This has led to forearm amputation in one previous case.

In regard to some of the technical aspects of the microsurgery, some size discrepancy, for instance, taking a 2-mm circumflex scapular artery and suturing it into a 3- to 4-mm distal brachial artery, is manageable. We can work with 1.5:1, even up to 2:1 size discrepancies with good patency rates, particularly with the larger vessels.

Dr. Zubowicz

I would like to make a point about the timing of coverage. I think perhaps a more conventional way of managing this would have been to do the revascularization with a vein graft and then treat the wound expectantly until the tissues had declared themselves. A delayed reconstruction follows either with a skin/fascia flap or a muscle flap with a skin graft.

I am concerned about doing a vascular reconstruction in an open, potentially contaminated wound, and whether or not it should be covered immediately. It is my opinion that it should not be immediately closed if an autogenous graft is used. I think you can adequately protect that type of exposed vascular graft by covering with physiologic dressings. That allows you more than adequate time for the situation to stabilize and then provide coverage in a semiurgent fashion rather than an emergent fashion.

Dr. French

Another approach might be to use a Gortex graft with immediate flap coverage. This would also obviate the need for a vein graft donor site. However, I would favor the elegant plan used in this case.

Dr. Grotting

Those are excellent points, and I would agree that there are very few indications for doing emergency free flaps. The only ones in my mind are where there are critical segmental vascular repairs where the price of being wrong is really quite high. In this situation, we had already had a failed saphenous vein graft. We felt that we had one solution that had to work. In terms of treating tissues expectantly, we knew that we were going to have enough soft tissue loss to have inadequate local tissues to repair or to cover the median nerve and the vascular repairs. So we were already committed to a distant tissue transfer, be it a pedicle flap or a free flap. One can't always be certain of the amount of debridement required, but to treat the wound in the fashion of Godina and debride it as one would a tumor back to fresh, normal tissues. I think one can be pretty certain that the debridement would be adequate.

DR. FRENCH

How far postinjury did you do this?

DR. GROTTING

Four hours.

DR. STAHL

One other point I would like to bring up is the aggressive use of fasciotomy in an ischemic upper extremity. Fasciotomy in this setting necessitates opening all muscle compartments in the forearm and hand as necessary. Failure to do this results in a salvaged upper extremity that is a nonfunctional one. I always perform a fasciotomy in electrical injuries, crush injuries, and prolonged ischemia. It is mostly a matter of clinical judgment. I agree with you, Dr. Grotting, that in a situation where we're going to have a compromised upper extremity, I would not look to the opposite arm for my reconstructive solution.

DR. MOSES

I would like to add a historical note. In an emergency situation this flap is a brilliant solution to a complex series of needs for this type of wound. In the early days of microsurgery, when Dr. Jim May of Boston first described the latissimus dorsi free flap, his preferred technique was to include a "T" of subscapular artery and to inset the flap with two end-to-end anastomoses exactly as you have done now. In those days, this was done before we had all realized the simple utility of an end-to-end microanastomosis. That technique was subsequently dropped. Here, in an emergency situation, you have rediscovered something that has been dropped from current usage.

DR. STAHL

Do you recall if you had any noninvasive studies postoperatively, segmental pressures, pulse-volume recordings compared to the opposite extremity?

DR. GROTTING

No, we did not do any sophisticated measurements like that, but I can tell you there were no palpable pulses at the wrist preoperatively. These returned immediately after revascularization and have persisted in the period of postoperative follow-up.

REFERENCES

1. Harii K, Ohmori K, Ohmori S. Successful clinical transfer of ten free flaps by microvascular anastomoses. Plast Reconstr Surg 1974;53:259.

2. Mathes S, Alpert B. Free skin and composite flaps. In: Green DP, editor. Operative hand surgery 1988;27:1151–1213.

3. Godina M. The tailored latissimus dorsi free flap. Plast Reconstr Surg 1987;80:304–306.

4. Coleman JJ, Sultan MR. The bipedicled osteocutaneous scapula flap. A new subscapular system free flap. Plast Reconstr Surg 1991;87:682.

5. Lister GD. Emergency free flaps. In: Green DP editor. Operative hand surgery. 1988;2:1127–1149.

6. Bonawitz SC, Schnarrs RH, Rosenthal AI, Rogers GK, Newton ED. Free tissue transfer in elderly patients. Plast Reconstr Surg 1991;87:1074–1079.

EXTENSIVE HAND COVERAGE WITH THE REVERSED RADIAL FOREARM FLAP

JAMES C. GROTTING AND CARL C. ASKREN

THE PROBLEM

The patient was a 21-year-old woman who sustained an injury to the dorsum of her nondominant hand in a motor vehicle accident. Her hand was outside the vehicle when it rolled over, resulting in loss of skin and extensor tendons and fracture of all four finger metacarpals (Figure 8.1). Her initial care included surgical debridement and pinning of her metacarpals (Figure 8.2). The dorsal wrist ligaments were also repaired. Several debridements were required to achieve a clean wound. Consultation was received at 8 days postinjury.

INTRODUCTION

Injuries of the hand and forearm range from the more superficial wounds, such as partial-thickness burns, to upper extremity amputations. Each injury presents its own reconstructive challenges. The goal in treating upper extremity wounds is to achieve primary wound healing. If this cannot be accomplished, problems develop with tissue in wounds that are left open

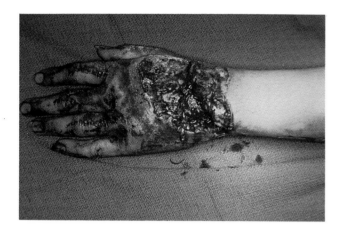

Figure 8.1. Dorsal hand injury resulting from a motor vehicle accident. Note soft tissue loss involving extensor tendons as well as skin and subcutaneous fat.

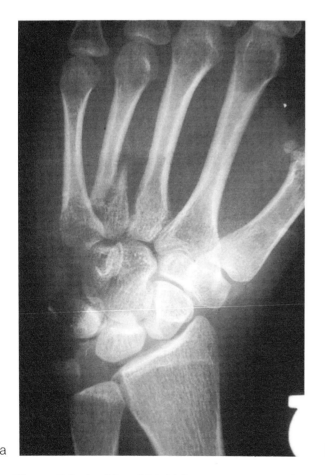

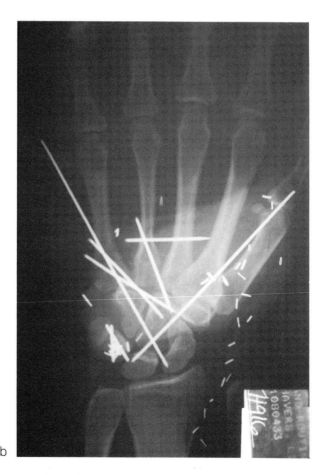

a   b

Figure 8.2. (a, b). (a) Initial x-ray appearance demonstrating loss of the dorsal cortex of all four finger metacarpals as well as fractures. (b) Postreduction appearance.

following injury. Desiccation of bone and tendon can occur even with the best of care. Granulation tissue is always contaminated. Soft tissue edema contributes to fibrosis and friability of vessels. With primary wound closure, there is a minimum of inflammation that would otherwise result in edema, joint stiffness, and adhesions. How the soft tissue is managed thus becomes fundamental to quality care of the wound.

A distally based radial forearm flap was selected for coverage. The presence of both radial and ulnar arteries was verified by palpation, and an Allen's test was used to confirm dominance of the ulnar system. A pattern of the defect was made, and this was marked on the volar forearm about 10 cm proximal to the wrist crease. The cephalic vein was also marked. Dissection was performed under tourniquet control. The flap was raised from proximal to distal, sparing the radial nerve and including a branch of the cephalic vein. The flap was passed through a subcutaneous tunnel created to connect with the primary defect, and then the flap was inset (Figure 8.3a,b). The donor site required a small skin graft.

The postoperative course was uneventful. Initial healing of the island flap was satisfactory (Figure 8.4). Extensor reconstruction was performed by Dr. Donald H. Lee approximately 6 months following injury (Figure 8.5a,b). The final appearance of the donor site is shown in Figure 8.6.

Anatomy

The radial forearm flap has become a common solution for upper extremity wounds, not only as a free tissue transfer, but also as a local flap. As an island flap, it may be based either proximally or distally, depending on the location of the primary defect. Distally based, it lends itself well to coverage of the dorsum of the hand for injuries commonly sustained in the overturning vehicle.[1] Since the hand and fingers receive their blood supply mainly from the ulnar artery, a modified Allen's test will demonstrate whether retrograde flow is satisfactory to supply the distally based flap.

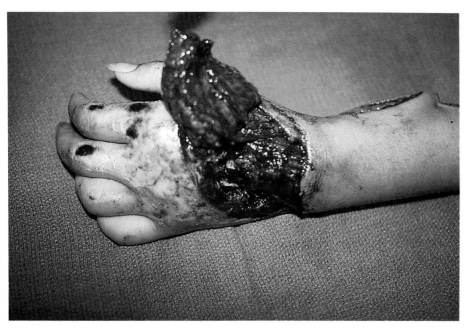

a

Figure 8.3. (a, b) (a) A reversed radial forearm flap was harvested, rotated, and tunneled subcutaneously through the "snuffbox." (b) Intraoperative appearance following inset.

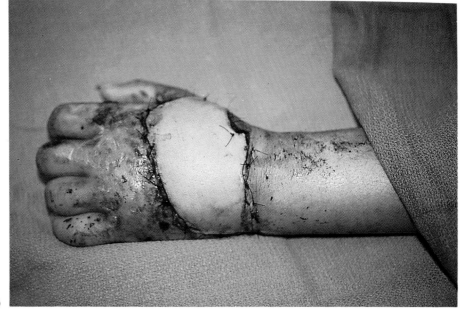

b

Figure 8.4. The healed flap prior to extensor tendon reconstruction.

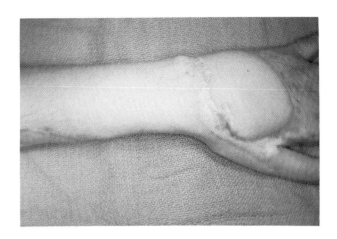

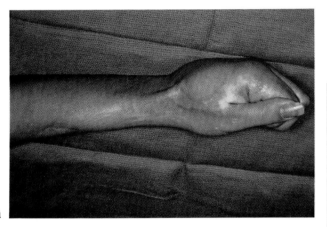

a

Figure 8.5. Final postoperative result following extensor tendon reconstruction demonstrating flexion (a) and extension (b).

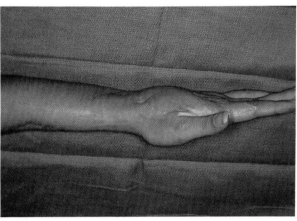

b

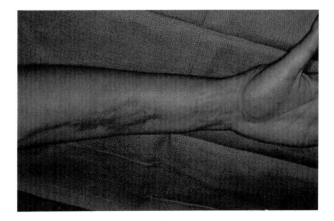

Figure 8.6. Final appearance of donor site (no revisions).

Most of the palmar forearm skin is supplied by the radial artery, so that a flap can be planned almost anywhere on the forearm, provided the perforating vessels from the artery are maintained. The perforators lie over the artery within the intermuscular septum between the bracyhioradialis and the flexor carpi radialis. The radial artery is generally approached underneath the forearm fascia from either side of this septum.

The flap has been criticized for its donor defect, but in selected cases, it can be used such that the donor site is closed primarily, or with only a small skin graft that can easily be revised.

Technique

Using an x-ray film template, an exact pattern of the defect is constructed. The pattern is transferred to the forearm at a sufficient length proximal to the wrist flexion crease so that the flap can easily be draped into the defect. This is usually about 10 cm. The pattern does not have to be centered directly over the radial artery, but it should be oriented so that the radial-most edge of the flap (once it is inset) is closest to the pedicle.

Dissection of the flap is facilitated by application of a pneumatic tourniquet and with the use of loupe magnification. The flap is incised at its periphery down through the fascia. The fascia is elevated off the flexor carpi radialis and brachioradialis until the intermuscular septum is reached (Figure 8.7). The artery and its venae comitantes are identified and surrounded. Perforating branches to the fascia are readily visualized. Deeper branches to adjacent muscles are divided after bipolar cautery or the application of microclips. To accomplish this, the artery must be dissected distally to the level of the wrist, and an extension of the skin incision must be made directly over the radial artery (Figure 8.8). The radial artery can then be ligated and divided proximally.

During the dissection, if a superficial vein can easily be preserved within the flap, this may be done. Because of the presence of valves, however, its precise contribution to venous drainage is not known. The venous drainage of the flap must be retrograde through the venae comitantes or a

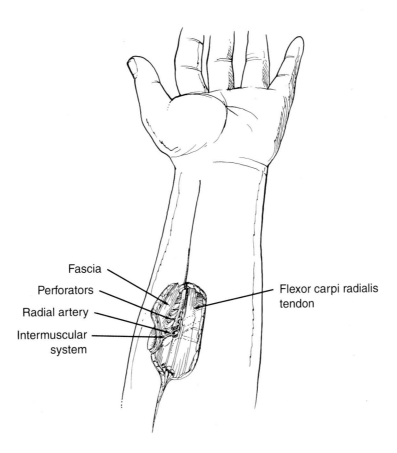

Fascia

Perforators

Radial artery

Intermuscular
system

Flexor carpi radialis
tendon

Figure 8.7. Flap design showing preservation of peritenon and perforators passing through the intermuscular septum.

superficial vein. This is possible either because a pressure head exists sufficient to render the valves incompetent, or because flow occurs through a circuitous route via veins bridging the comitant veins, thus bypassing the valves.[2]

A subcutaneous tunnel of sufficient size to accommodate the flap is made from the donor site to the primary defect. This is performed at the level of the fascia to protect the sensory branches of the radial nerve. Inset is carried out with half-buried horizontal mattress sutures using 4-0 nylon. Tendon reconstruction may be either carried out simultaneously or delayed until primary healing has occurred. Elevation of the hand diminishes postoperative edema and aids venous outflow.

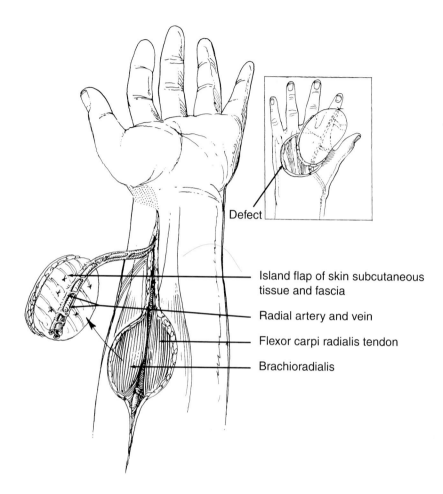

Defect

Island flap of skin subcutaneous tissue and fascia

Radial artery and vein

Flexor carpi radialis tendon

Brachioradialis

Figure 8.8. Concept of distally based reversed radial forearm flap for dorsal hand coverage.

Discussion

Management of patients with traumatic injuries of the upper extremity should follow the principles of management of any trauma patient. Attention should be directed toward diagnosing any life-threatening injuries and treating them first. The extremity then takes on a lower priority. The exceptions are exsanguinating hemorrhage from the limb or limb devascularization. Myonecrosis begins after about 4 hours. A fasciotomy should be performed to avoid a compartment syndrome if the ischemia is prolonged.

Patients should also be hemodynamically stable. Multiple traumas, prolonged anesthesia, and massive transfusions are associated with increased complications.

Acute traumatic wounds are usually contaminated. To prevent infection, untidy wounds must be rendered tidy by debridement. This, along with intravenous antibiotics, better prepares the wounds to resist infection.

Some authors advocate aggressive initial debridement.[3,4] However, in situations where radical debridement may destroy critical specialized structures that are potentially salvageable, it may be wise to retain questionable tissue and remove it in a subsequent debridement. A "second look" at 24 to 48 hours is then warranted, at which time the wound may be covered. If doubt still remains and further debridement is required, the chance of infection rises. Under circumstances of heavy contamination, the wound may need to be skin grafted where possible after the final debridement and flap reconstruction deferred until after the wound is healed. With improved flap reliability, this management technique has become a rare event.

Flap coverage can and should be accomplished at the earliest practical time in order to achieve the goal of primary wound healing. Early wound closure has been defined as closure within 72 hours of injury.[5] With aggressive debridement, tissue can be transferred at the time of the initial surgery. This has been referred to as *emergency* free tissue transfer. Briedenbach[6] has nicely detailed when to use emergency free tissue transfer based on the extent of debridement, bacterial load, fracture type and location, and the presence of exposed vital structures. We agree with Acland[7] that waiting 2 to 3 days until the patient, the doctor, and the wound are all adequately prepared for a major procedure has not adversely affected the final outcome.

Immediate or early reconstruction of vessels, plate fixation, bone grafts, tendon repair, joint replacement, and grafts of nerve or tendon provides a psychological benefit to the patients, reduced total hospital time, and economic benefits for the community because of the potential for earlier return to work or occupational retraining.

Skin grafting has been traditionally indicated for wounds that cannot be approximated primarily. However, because of the complexity of the underlying structures in the hand, this method of wound closure is useful only in the most superficial of avulsion injuries. In severe injuries of the hand, the reconstructive effort must furnish satisfactory coverage of the bone and tendons, with vascularized tissue and preferably subcutaneous fat to provide gliding surfaces that do not restrict motion. Under skin grafts, tendons do not glide, bone cannot be satisfactorily covered, and sensibility cannot be provided for.

Flaps, on the other hand, have their own blood supply, are more durable, allow tendon gliding, can provide sensibility, and reduce myofibroblast wound contracture. With the range of functional losses that may occur and the variety of reconstructive options, considerations for flap coverage of the upper extremity should be based on reconstructive needs. An adequate assessment based on examination of the wound under anesthesia is essential. Exposed structures such as bones, tendons, nerves, and vessels all require consideration of both skin and fat for coverage.

Although many reconstructive procedures are performed electively, the reconstructive surgeon may be called upon in the acute setting, and special needs must be addressed at that time.[3,4]

Millard has set forth an important aesthetic principle for replacing lost tissue: it should be replaced with tissue of like color and texture.[8] Local tissue can provide similar skin without creating a distant donor site, and it becomes the first choice when available. However, tissue in the upper extremity is not easily spared and must be transferred with great care to minimize donor site morbidity. Raising a local flap traumatizes an already injured limb, and the resultant wound can potentially impair function more than the original soft tissue defect. Also, local flaps are limited in size,[9] and in moderate to severe injuries there is generally insufficient local tissue. Distant pedicled flaps or free tissue transfer techniques are then required to accomplish reconstruction.

Larger wounds of the hand have been acutely covered with distant flaps. These flaps can achieve wound closure, but they carry with them certain disadvantages: a secondary procedure for division of the pedicle and inset is required, possible debulking procedures may be needed, and early motion may be cumbersome or impossible. Additional problems with distant flaps are that circumferential defects are difficult to cover, and young children or certain adults may not be compliant with positioning.

From the perspective of rehabilitation, the disadvantages are that the hand must be immobilized and dependent. This results in discomfort, chronic edema, and stiffness. If complete coverage can be accomplished in a single procedure, this will allow elevation of the extremity, better control of edema, and early hand therapy because there is no distant site of attachment.

Edema and venous congestion are the main problems seen after reversed radial forearm flap transfer. Not only is venous drainage necessarily via retrograde flow through the pedicle, but closing the secondary defect primarily may result in a constricting effect on the proximal forearm. This could potentially compromise venous and lymphatic outflow of the flap and hand. Including a superficial vein with the flap during its dissection may be helpful to assist in venous drainage.

For moderate-sized soft tissue defects of the hand, the distally based radial forearm island flap provides an excellent means of coverage. A sufficient skin paddle can be raised without the disadvantages encountered with distant flaps, such as immobility, dependency, and hygiene. Soft tissue coverage of larger and more complex wounds can be achieved with free tissue transfer. Additional reconstructive requirements for bone or tendon may also be met with this type of procedure. Free flaps are preferably performed early, generally within the first 48 to 72 hours, to achieve the goal of primary wound healing.

ROUNDTABLE DISCUSSION

DR. GROTTING

In this case, a young woman with a very aesthetic abdominal wall was very anxious to return to work as fast as possible. In developing a reconstructive plan, we considered very strongly the use of a groin flap, but I felt that due to the size of the area and the volume of skin available in the forearm, I could transfer sufficient skin from the forearm in a single stage to supply all the missing soft tissue over the dorsum of the hand and very nearly be able to close the donor defect on the forearm primarily. We were able to close the donor site about 80%, skin grafting the remainder, knowing that we would be back in this patient for extensor tendon reconstruction. At that time the remaining skin graft might be able to be excised.

DR. TOTH

It is very refreshing for me to see that every problem in Birmingham, Alabama, doesn't require a microsurgical solution. In this case there were many potential microsurgical solutions. You used a reliable, regional flap that allowed a one-stage procedure without a distant secondary donor site. I would like to commend you on the elegance of the planning of this procedure in terms of being able to primarily close your donor site, as well as provide the appropriate coverages necessary.

DR. ELLIOTT

I, too, think that management of this case was done well. I think I probably would have used a free tissue transfer, because I think that despite the fact the donor site was mostly closed, you still harvested a significant amount of tissue from an already injured extremity and that has its drawbacks.

We think of the abdominal tissues as being thick, with a good bit of fat. In a thin patient, abdominal tissue can replace the hand dorsum fairly well. This patient was thin—and you mentioned the groin flap was a possibility, but any variation around the groin or lower abdomen would have provided fairly thin coverage.

Another thought would have been the dorsalis pedis flap with extensor tendons. That donor defect is not usually one I put very high on the list, but is something to think about. There are other donor sites: Lateral arm flap from the opposite arm, scapular flap or scapular fascia flap, even a temporal parietal fascial flap—all in a young person are good donor sites and provide appropriate replacement tissue.

Dr. Zubowicz

I find myself in the unusual position of being in agreement with Dr. Elliott. I think that in most circumstances, an ipsilateral radial forearm flap doesn't allow primary closure. For coverage of the dorsum of the hand, particularly in the thin patient, I have had very good luck using the groin flap. I think, generally, it is not too cumbersome, it does give you a small amount of fat, so that when the orthopedic surgeon or the plastic surgeon comes back to do tendon grafting at a later time, they have the opportunity for tendon excursion through the fat.

One other point has to do with timing of the coverage. I don't see any compelling reason to charge in and get things covered up. It is my attitude that physiologic dressings generally can provide the necessary care until the tissues have stabilized. I think that it is imperative during this period that hand therapy be begun immediately and mobilization of the wrist, fingers, etc., has to be done while the wound is still open. Then, after the tissues again have declared themselves, go ahead and perform the free tissue transfer. My choice is the free groin flap unless there are mitigating circumstances.

Dr. Moses

Regarding choice of donor site, I think Drs. Zubowicz and Elliott may have forgotten that the dorsum of the hand is also an aesthetically significant unit and that, while attention must be paid to the aesthetics of the donor site scar, the recipient site is also important in this case. The aesthetic quality of coverage from pedicled forearm skin is much superior to either a skin graft on a fascial flap or to a thick biscuit-like lower abdominal skin flap. My only concern in harvesting tissues from the injured extremity would have been to be sure of the vascularity of the forearm flap via a preoperative Allen's test.

Dr. Grotting

These have been good points and I think that a discussion of donor site was the major issue in this patient. This was a young woman who spent time at the beach wearing a bathing suit. I think what you need to keep in mind is that, no matter how elegant a reconstruction you are able to do on the dorsum of the hand, there will always be significant scarring on that extremity. My feeling was trying to limit the donor scarring to that extremity was better than creating a secondary scar somewhere else. I don't think that a scar on the back as in the case of the scapular flap, or even a scar on the groin, would necessarily have ended up with a better aesthetic situation than I ended up with here.

DR. FRENCH

I still feel that it is easier to cover a scar in the groin with a swimsuit than it is to cover a forearm scar. If the groin flap is too thick, secondary suctioning can easily contour it.

DR. GROTTING

The issue regarding extensor tendon reconstruction is a good one. Under ideal circumstances, if a wound has stabilized and can be covered in the first 4 to 5 days postoperatively when there is not a lot of hospital contamination, then one could consider either primary extensor tendon reconstruction or the placement of Hunter tendon rods at least to create tunnels for secondary reconstruction. We elected to defer tendon reconstruction until we had ideal circumstances.

DR. TOTH

Have you ever done secondary tendon grafting under a free fascial flap?

DR. GROTTING

That is a good question, and that is the reason we felt that temporoparietal fascia in this circumstance would not have given us an adequate gliding bed, although we would have been able to achieve a healed wound. Going back and trying to create gliding surfaces over a very scarred wound bed consisting of the dorsal wrist capsule and a fascial flap, which in my experience tends to atrophy to extreme thinness, would not have been as ideal a circumstance as having a layer of fat and normal skin. Although, admittedly, the biplanar temporoparietal fascial flap which includes both the superficial and deep temporal fascia as two separate layers has been used for exactly this purpose (i.e., sandwich tendon grafting).

DR. ELLIOTT

One option we haven't discussed is the pedicled groin or transfer abdominal flaps. One drawback to the flaps is persistent edema resulting from dependent positioning. Also complete hand therapy is delayed until the pedicle is divided.

REFERENCES

1. Mehrotra ON, Crabb DJM. The pattern of hand injury sustained in the overturning motor vehicle. Hand 1979;11:321–328.

2. Timmons MJ. The vascular basis of the radial forearm reconstruction. Plast Reconstr Surg 1986;77:80–92.

3. Lister GD, Scheker LR. Emergency free flaps to the upper extremity. J Hand Surg 1988;13A:22–28.

4. Lister GD. Emergency free flaps. In: Green DP, editor. Operative hand surgery. 1988;2:1127–1149.

5. Godina M. Early microsurgical reconstruction of complex trauma of the extremities. Plast Reconstr Surg 1986;78:285–292.

6. Breidenbach WC III. Emergency free tissue transfer for reconstruction of upper extremity wounds. Clin Plast Surg 1989;16:505–514.

7. Acland, RD. Refinements in lower extremity free flap surgery. Clin Plast Surg 1980;17:733–744.

8. Millard DR Jr. Principalization of Plastic Surgery. Boston: Little, Brown and Company, 1986.

9. Strausch B, Vasconez LO, Findley-Hall EJ, editors. Grabb's encyclopedia of Flaps. Vol. II. Boston: Little, Brown and Company, 1990.

5

DECISION MAKING
IN
ABDOMINAL
RECONSTRUCTION

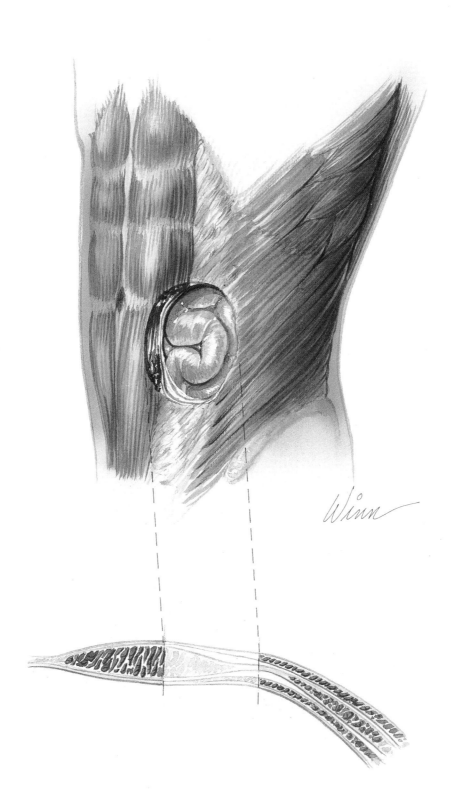

Reconstruction of Full-Thickness Defects of the Abdominal Wall

Vincent N. Zubowicz

The Problem

A 62-year-old diabetic and alcoholic patient developed synergistic gangrene of the scrotum that spread rapidly across the perineum and lower abdomen. The source of the infection remains unclear. The urologist began debridement of all involved tissue, which resulted, after several operations, in entire loss of the scrotum, perineum, and lower abdominal wall. The abdominal loss was complete from the umbilicus to the pubis.

After the infection was controlled surgically and medically, the patient was stabilized and return of multiple system organ failure was corrected. The intestines were kept within the abdominal cavity by dressing packs which were changed frequently. After 2 weeks, there were enough adhesions of the bowel to itself as well as to the walls of the peritoneal cavity to prevent evisceration. Granulation tissue soon covered the exposed intestines, the shaft of the penis, the testicles, and perineum (Figures 9.1 and 9.2).

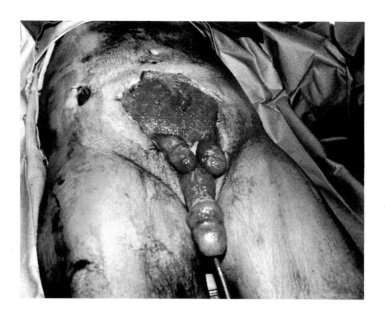

Figure 9.1. Full-thickness loss of abdominal wall as a result of necrotizing fasciitis.

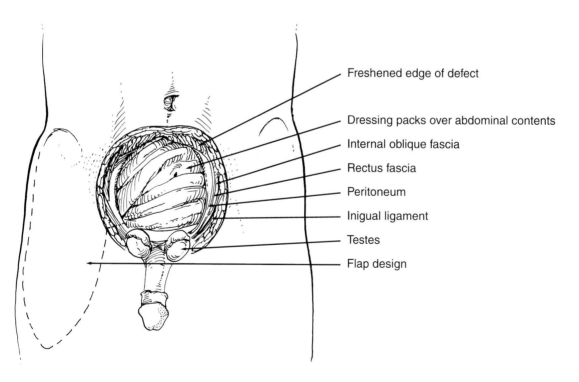

Freshened edge of defect

Dressing packs over abdominal contents

Internal oblique fascia

Rectus fascia

Peritoneum

Inigual ligament

Testes

Flap design

Figure 9.2. Illustration of full-thickness loss of abdominal wall including skin, muscle, fascia, and peritoneum.

INTRODUCTION

Reconstruction of the abdomen ranges from simple to exceptionally complex, depending upon the defect. The abdominal wall provides structural support for the abdomen and confinement of the contents of the peritoneal cavity. This is the domain of the abdominal musculature and fascia. This is a dynamic unit partially composed of static structural components.

The abdominal wall must also have skin covering. Roughly 10% of the skin surface area of the body is found on the abdominal wall. The skin provides enough elasticity for flexion and extension of the trunk.

This discussion will be confined to total abdominal wall reconstruction. That is, we will be looking at defects that result from loss of skin, subcutaneous tissue, muscle, and fascia. Split-thickness grafts remain the mainstay for skin loss with the other components intact. Fascia and prosthetic meshes work well when abdominal structural integrity is lost but skin coverage is adequate.

It is certainly possible, and occasionally highly advisable, to provide skin coverage by way of a split-thickness graft without immediately addressing musculofascial support. This results in a closed wound at the expense of an obligatory hernia. In critically ill patients, staged reconstruction is indicated. When the wound is controlled and the patient is stable, elective reconstruction of all components can be undertaken. In elderly and disabled patients, life with a large hernia may be the best compromise.

PATIENT MANAGEMENT

Initial management was directed at accomplishing a closed wound with the least risk to the desperately ill patient. This was accomplished by a thin split-thickness graft applied to all open areas. The grafts were successful at closing the wound, but left the patient with thin coverage over the testicles and bowel.

Several months later, after the patient had returned home and regained a measure of strength, elective reconstruction was planned at his

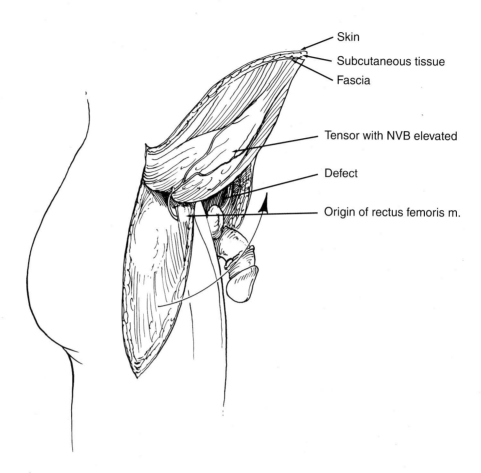

Skin
Subcutaneous tissue
Fascia

Tensor with NVB elevated

Defect

Origin of rectus femoris m.

Figure 9.3. (a, b). (a) Tensor fasciae latae flap mobilized as a pedicle or island flap for full-thickness coverage of lower one-half of the abdomen.

insistence. It should be remembered that he could live, albeit with significant handicap, with the coverage provided by the skin graft. However, a large lower abdominal hernia would ultimately develop.

Reconstruction involved reestablishment of fascial integrity of the abdominal wall followed by skin and soft-tissue coverage. The split-thickness graft was peeled away from the loops of bowel. This is an easy dissection. Freshened edges of the abdominal fascia were exposed for reconstruction.

A tensor fasciae latae island flap was chosen for reconstruction (Figure 9.3a). Because the defect existed within the lower half of the abdomen, this flap was expected to fulfill the tissue needs without difficulty. The fas-

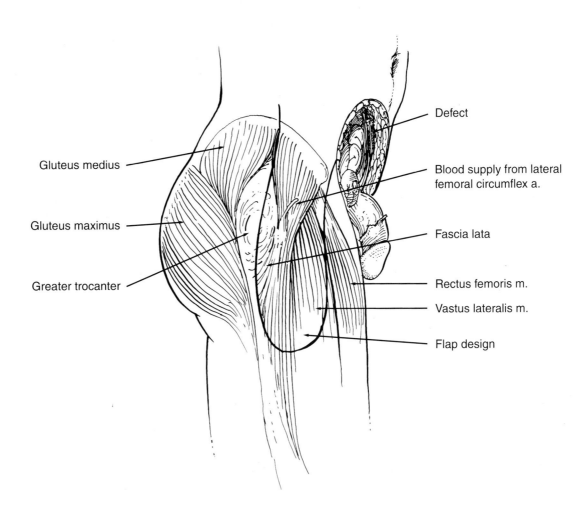

(b) Tensor fasciae latae flap based on the lateral femoral circumflex vessel entering the flap approximately 10 cm below the anterior superior iliac spine.

cia of the lateral thigh reconstituted abdominal wall integrity without the use of synthetic mesh. The skin carried with the flap provided coverage (Figure 9.4).

Convalescence was complicated by seroma formation both beneath the flap and within the primarily closed donor site. This was managed on an outpatient basis by repeated syringe aspiration, although 2 months passed before all drainage ceased. The ultimate result was satisfactory (Figure 9.5a,b).

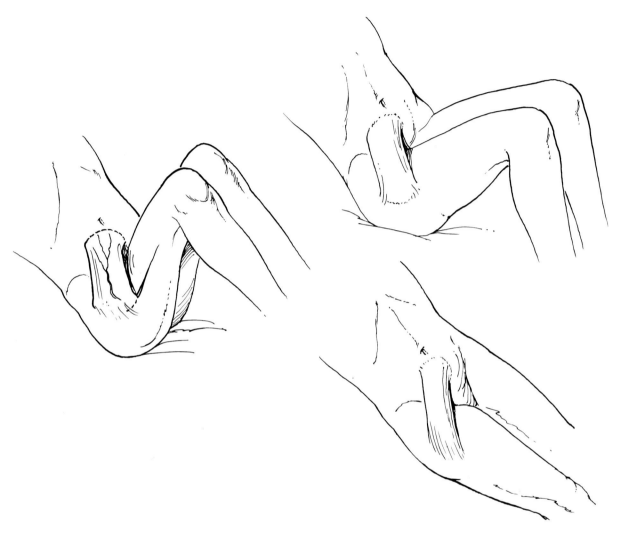

Figure 9.4. Abdominal flexion to allow for tension-free closure of abdominal wall defect.

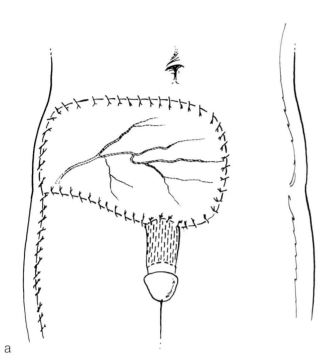

a

Figure 9.5. (a, b). (a) Graphic representation of reconstruction of lower abdomen with tensor fasciae latae muscle and fascia flap. (b) Final result of reconstruction with tensor fasciae latae myofasciocutaneous flap without the use of synthetic mesh.

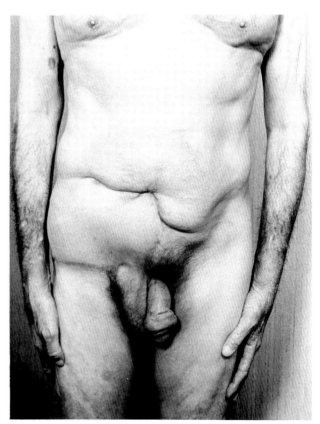

b

Anatomy

Dissection of the tensor fasciae latae as a free tissue transfer or as a pedicle flap is simple and rapid. The flap is based on the lateral circumflex vessels coursing medial to lateral. The pedicle enters the tensor fasciae muscle on its anteromedial edge 6 to 8 cm below the anterior superior iliac spine. It can be found under the hood of the rectus femoris muscle just deep to a thick band of fascia.

The entire flap is designed with the marking pen and can carry usable fascia to below the knee. The flap is developed as an island or a peninsula depending upon the requirements for reconstruction. The initial incision can be carried to the fascia with impunity, as the pedicle lies deep to it. The fascia is incised quickly, except near the pedicle, and elevated by blunt dissection. Small areolar perforators on the deep surface may produce annoying but insignificant bleeding.

The flap is elevated from the distal to the proximal end until the region of the vascular pedicle is reached. Here the posterior side of the muscle is reflected anteriorally and the pedicle is identified from the deep side. With the vessels now in view, division of the fascia on the anterior side of the flap is easily performed, and the flap can be converted safely into a true island flap. Note that the arc of rotation, determined by the level of entry of the pedicle into the flap, is 6 cm or so below the anterior superior iliac spine. In predicting the capabilities of an individual flap, one should be cognizant of the geometry of the tethering pedicle.

In most circumstances, the donor site can be closed primarily. Problems with wound separation at the junction of the proximal closure to the adjacent island flap are common because of tension associated with the meeting of two suture lines. If tension is too great to allow primary closure, a split-thickness skin graft is applied.

Discussion

Reconstruction of the abdominal wall may be approached in a variety of ways, depending upon the defect involved and the overall health of the patient. As stated above, fascial defects alone are managed nicely in most cases by synthetic mesh. Skin loss with preservation of musculofascial support calls for skin grafts, local skin flaps, or skin expansion. In this chapter, the discussion will be limited to full-thickness loss of portions of the abdominal wall.

Most commonly used are musculofascial flaps from the thigh.[1-4] Both the rectus femoris and the tensor fasciae latae flaps can be rotated on their pedicles for composite tissue replacement. However, for defects that extend above the umbilicus and approach the xiphoid, their lengths are unpredictable. More often than not, the repairs in this region are disturbingly tight if accomplishable at all.

Whether or not these flaps of the upper thigh reach depends on the length of the patient's thigh relative to the abdominal height. Mobilization of the donor arteries and veins to their origin may give several additional centimeters. Usually, the repair of the upper abdomen is a compromise or unobtainable.

Additional length or more favorable orientation may be achieved by detaching the flaps and transferring them as free tissue transfers.[5] The superior epigastric vessels dissected below the costal margin provide arterial flow and venous drainage, although the dissection is tedious. Free tissue transfer of this type allows much more satisfactory reconstruction of the upper abdomen, notwithstanding the additional technical difficulties.

Other flaps are available for reconstruction if the operating microscope is to be employed. The latissimus can provide a large surface area, although no formal fascial layer is transferred with it. In my experience with only two cases, the integrity of the abdominal wall with significant herniation persisted, even though no synthetic mesh was used as a fascial substitute under the free muscle transfer.

Nevertheless, the preferred flap is the tensor fasciae latae because of the thick and broad section of tough fascia available. The blood supply is predictable and easily dissected,[6] and donor morbidity is tolerable.

It is acceptable and possibly preferable to provide structural integrity with synthetic mesh[7] and then cover it with vascularized tissue. If mesh is to be used, skin grafts placed on granulation tissue that has percolated through the interstices of the mesh for coverage are doomed to failure. They may provide adequate temporary coverage but in time will need to be replaced by vascularized skin. The mesh has now become exposed and contaminated and should be replaced at the same time.

Delayed coverage of mesh with vascularized tissue is also not a good idea. When mesh is chosen as a fascial substitute, immediate vascularized coverage should be performed. Bacterial colonization in the interstices of this foreign substance will result in chronic sinuses or frank abscess. Immediate coverage will combat this.

All suture lines must be buried in vascularized tissue. Synthetic mesh, even when it is to be covered immediately by vascularized tissue, should not remain in contact with a fresh suture line if a stoma has been closed at the time of abdominal wall reconstruction. Omentum or serosa of uninjured bowel should be insinuated between the suture line and the abdominal wall reconstruction.

Soft tissue expansion as a prelude to abdominal wall reconstruction makes good sense if the anatomy allows it. The expanders should be placed when abdominal wounds are controlled, and any stomas are drained and sealed. The risk of infection is obviously greater with open wounds or nearby stomas.

At the time of reconstruction, all bowel anastomoses would be buried under omentum or loops of bowel. A synthetic mesh (Prolene is best) would be placed to reconstitute fascial integrity. The expanded skin would then be advanced to close the skin defect over the fascia. Obviously, wound healing problems could become manifest all the way into the peritoneal cavity when this method of reconstruction is employed.

At present, there is probably no one preferred method for total abdominal reconstruction. The tensor fasciae latae is the best when only the lower abdomen is considered. However, when defects are higher (and they usually are), free tissue transfer may be required for the best "fit."

In any reconstruction, the wound should always be closed before total reconstruction is begun. A skin graft will provide coverage and sterilize the area. Later, the graft can be easily removed and formal reconstruction with any of the techniques mentioned above can be performed.

Roundtable Discussion

Dr. Zubowicz

Immediate reconstruction of full-thickness defects is permissible after resections of tumor. It is contraindicated after trauma or infection until the wound has stabilized. By this I mean that the wound is clean, all remaining tissue is viable and healthy, and inflammation has subsided. In the case of this particular patient, stability of the wound was accomplished by a split-thickness skin graft. Only after the inflammation had subsided was definite full-thickness reconstruction undertaken.

The choice of tensor fasciae latae was easy in this case. First of all, the wound was below the umbilicus. The tensor fasciae latae does well with these wounds as it is less reliable in the upper half of the abdomen. Second, the condition of the femoral vessels was good, promising a healthy lateral circumflex blood supply to the flap. Finally, donor morbidity was minimal in this patient.

Other considered options included the rectus femoris—not a particularly good choice for reasons of donor morbidity and paucity of good fascia. Various free tissue transfers, including the latissimus, are certainly options. They lack, however, the tough fascia of the tensor fasciae latae, which is crucial to the integrity of the abdominal fascial reconstruction. Furthermore, the tensor fasciae latae may be used as a free tissue transfer (I have done this for *upper* abdominal reconstruction) to facilitate its orientation in the wound. This was unnecessary in this case.

Dr. Stahl

The tensor fasciae latae was the correct choice. Remember that the habitus of the patient, the length of the thigh, and the position of the wound on the abdomen all determine the utility of the tensor fasciae latea as a rotation flap. Careful measurement and planning are required to avoid a flap that is under excess tension or even is incapable of closing the wound.

Dr. Elliott

The fascia overlying the tensor fasciae muscle and the rectus femoris is continuous, running from the femoral canal laterally to the septum between the hamstrings and the vastus lateralis. This sheet is nourished by musculocutaneous perforators from both the rectus femoris muscle and the tensor fasciae latae muscle. This allows for this *entire* sheet of fascia to be elevated on either muscle.

I also agree that the reliability of this transfer falters above the umbilicus. As Dr. Stahl correctly points out, the habitus and thigh length are critical determinants.

Dr. Moses

Dr. Zubowicz is no genius for choosing the tensor fasciae latae. After all, it includes exactly those elements that were missing in the abdominal wall of the patient—fascia, an intervening layer of fat, and vascularized skin. As a matter of fact, in this case there was really no other legitimate choice.

I would restate Dr. Elliott's point about harvesting extensions of fascia, but with slightly different emphasis. With full-thickness wounds, the skin can be easily advanced several centimeters while the fascia cannot. The tensor fasciae latae (or rectus femoris) can be designed with a smaller skin paddle sitting atop a very broad expanse of fascia. Combined with the opposite tensor fasciae latae, the flaps together can fill defects of a considerable size.

Dr. Stahl

I disagree with the idea that the tensor fasciae latae replaces just what is missing. Patients should be informed that this fascia is not contractile and is unlike the muscle that has been lost. They may experience a bulge that mimics a hernia even with successful myofascial transfer.

Dr. Grotting

I concur with the consensus regarding reconstruction of the abdominal wall *above* the umbilicus. In the patient with very long thighs, I have used one or both rectus femoris muscles to reconstruct the abdominal wall up to the xiphoid.

Dr. McKinnon

For those where the tensor fasciae latae is not long enough to reach the epigastrium, positioning the patient in semi-Fowler's position may allow the flap to reach. Over a period of several days to several weeks, the abdomen is gradually extended until the flap is accommodated with the patient fully erect. Testimonially, it has worked for me (Figure 9.4).

DR. STAHL

I too have tried this with success. It is also a way to remove tension on the repair, even when the flaps will close the wound with the patient flat on the operating table.

DR. ZUBOWICZ

We all seem to agree on the utility of the tensor fasciae latae. I am disappointed, however, in the group's lack of imagination. What else would any of you consider?

DR. GROTTING

In the patient with short thighs, particularly if they are obese, these musculofascial flaps will not reach. Two options should be considered. The first is the rectus *abdominis* muscle from one side, with either a horizontal or vertical skin island to replace the upper abdominal area, combined with the opposite rectus *femoris* muscle or tensor fasciae latae to replace the lower abdominal area (Figure 9.6).

The second is an older technique described by Hershey and Butcher in the 1950s. They developed a rectangular flap from the lower quadrant and shifted all of this to the upper abdomen for reconstruction. The resulting lower abdominal defect was closed with techniques that we have all been discussing.

DR. ZUBOWICZ

That's interesting, Dr. Grotting, although I can't see you choosing something like that when an operating microscope will do. When do you use free tissue transfer?

DR. GROTTING

Free tissue transfer should be reserved for only those cases that can't be managed by the other local transfers we have discussed. Donor artery and recipient veins in the upper abdomen are not easy to find and use. Selection of the flap for transfer should bring in elements that will not only restore soft-tissue coverage but also manage the fascial integrity of the abdominal wall.

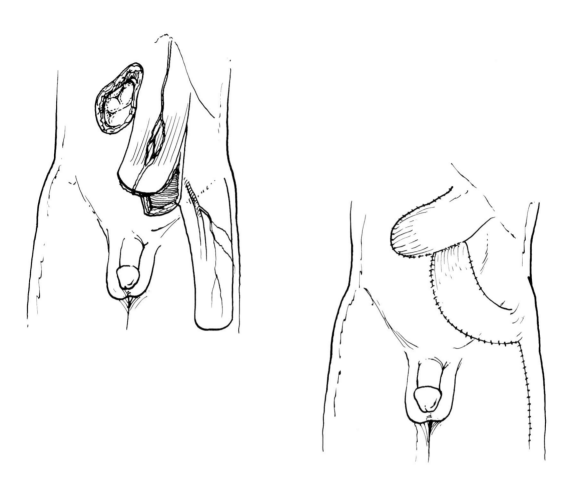

Figure 9.6. Tensor fasciae latae used to reconstruct donor defect created by rectus myocutaneous flap elevated for primary closure.

DR. ELLIOTT

When the rotation flap will not close wounds above the umbilicus, I favor the use of fascial reconstruction with a synthetic mesh covered by a free tissue transfer, my favorite being the latissimus dorsi.

DR. ZUBOWICZ

Dr. Elliott introduces synthetic mesh into the discussion. Is mesh really necessary? Does anyone use mesh with the tensor fasciae latae?

DR. ELLIOTT

Mesh is not required under a tensor fasciae latae flap. But I trust mesh more than I trust tensor fasciae latae particularly when it is covered by well-vascularized muscle. The mesh will be stable and solid. The fascia may tear, particularly later on.

DR. GROTTING

Under a free tissue transfer I favor the use of two layers of mesh with yet another layer of absorbable Vicryl mesh between the permanent mesh and the viscera. The gradual resorption of the Vicryl or Dexon diminishes the problems that sometimes occur as a result of erosion of the Prolene mesh through bowel. Mesh is not needed under a properly secured tensor fasciae latae flap.

I also believe that it is beneficial to preserve the innervation of both the tensor fasciae latae and the rectus femoris muscle when transposing for abdominal wall reconstruction. This will lend a measure of dynamic support to the abdominal wall.

DR. ZUBOWICZ

Maintain innervation to the tensor fasciae latae or rectus femoris? Does anyone else agree with this?

DR. STAHL

As far as preserving innervation to the tensor fasciae latae is concerned, I do not see how this would help. With the rectus there is some benefit, since much of the flap is muscular, but the tensor fasciae latae is mostly fascia, and I can't see innervation helping that at all.

Speaking of innervation and alternative ideas, another approach to the difficult epigastric zone is expansion of the latissimus in its native position. This is done slowly. When expansion is complete, the latissimus can be transferred as an innervated muscle.

DR. GROTTING

The advantage of maintaining innervation, even to the tensor fasciae latae, is the influence of a functional muscle tightening the fascia and maintaining it under tension during movement.

DR. ZUBOWICZ

The patient in the text was managed in stages. The open wound was first managed by wound toilet, then a split-thickness skin graft a week or so later, and finally conclusive reconstruction several months later. Was this prudent management or wasteful procrastination?

DR. STAHL

Management of the wound in stages was correct, particularly considering the infectious cause of the wound. It should be restated, however, that the immediate stage is unnecessary in tumor cases, where reconstruction can be planned of a healthy wound after resection.

DR. ELLIOTT

I agree with management in stages, and I would like to reemphasize your point about timing the removal of a split-thickness skin graft off bowel. I have tried this early, when there is still inflammation, and experienced a difficult time, with serosal tears and frank bowel tears resulting. If one waits at least 6 months, a flimsy layer of adventitia develops between the graft and the serosa of the bowel. It is then very easy to remove.

The patients may be anxious to complete the final reconstruction. However, it is important to wait for the inflammation to subside (6 months) before removing the graft. The operation will be hazardous if this rule is violated.

DR. ZUBOWICZ

I agree with Dr. Elliott. As a barometer of when the skin can be removed safely, I employ a type of "pinch" test. When the time is right for removal, one can pinch the skin graft and feel the bowl move away from the graft and the two sides of the skin graft come together.

A useful trick during removal is to inject a dilute lidocaine + epinephrine solution between the skin graft and the bowel (Figure 9.7). One can actually hydrodissect this plane. The plane becomes well defined and the epinephrine diminishes the oozing. I find the dissection very easy after this.

Now consider the problem of a stoma or fistula in the midst of an open composite wound of the abdomen. How do you deal with this? Can you close the stoma concurrently with abdominal wall reconstruction? Must you stage the reconstruction?

DR. ELLIOTT

In a patient with Crohn's Disease, I have to report an unsuccessful experience with closure of a fistula and immediate reconstruction of the lower abdomen.

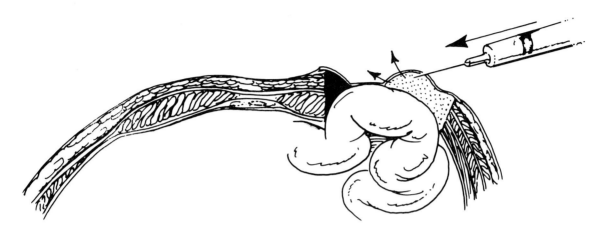

Figure 9.7. Hydrodissection of split-thickness skin graft from bowel wall facilitating sharp dissection.

After flap closure, there was continuous leakage. However, in this case the patient was quite debilitated and malnourished. I feel that the error was not in attempting fistula closure and reconstruction together but in attempting any surgery with the patient's state of nutrition.

Dr. Zubowicz

Dr. Elliott, your conclusions are right but with some adjustments. First of all, as you point out, the patient must be in good condition. This includes state of nutrition as well as condition of the wound. Then, and this is critically important, the suture line from repair or reanastomosis of bowel *must* be buried under omentum or serosa of adjacent bowel. The suture line should not be touching or exposed to the flap. Furthermore, the bowel should be electively prepped before surgery.

If these conditions cannot be met, then closure should precede abdominal reconstruction. In this scenario, the bowel would be repaired. The suture line would be buried beneath omentum or serosa. A skin graft would be applied to the exposed wound. Reconstruction of the abdomen would be undertaken 6 months or so later when all inflammation had subsided and the graft could be removed from the bowel easily.

Dr. Grotting

One must, of course, rule out causes for persistent fistula—distal obstruction, epithelialization of the track, or tumor. Unless you cover the fistula repair, it will invariably break down. You must cover it with a flap, omentum, or another loop of bowel.

DR. STAHL

I prefer to stage abdominal reconstruction in the presence of a fistula whenever possible. My philosophy is to keep things simple. Therefore, close the fistula. Wait. Then reconstruct the abdominal wall when the fistula is history.

DR. MCKINNON

Returning to the tensor fasciae latae and technical considerations, how do you deal with a circular defect in the abdomen by effectively closing it 360° without compromising blood supply to the distal tensor fasciae latae flap?

DR. STAHL

A technical problem involves securing the fascia of a transferred tensor fasciae latae or rectus myofascial flap at the proximal fascial insetting. Here one is dealing with the integrity of the repair versus overzealous suturing possibly compromising the vascular inflow/outflow. Suturing here should be done meticulously to avoid a postoperative hernia. This area worries me a lot.

DR. ZUBOWICZ

With the tensor fasciae latae, I carefully cut the fascia, leaving the areolar tissue between the fascia and the fat intact. I have done this several times and have not compromised the distal flap. The fascia can then be easily sutured into the defect end to end.

DR. MOSES

I suture circumferentially without cutting it, by overlapping the fascia of the flap with the cut edge.

DR. STAHL

If you can get the sutures into place, I see no problem with that. I prefer to get better control of the edge of the fascia by carefully cutting it. Blind sutures into the areolar layer, whether the fascia is cut or not, may compromise the blood supply.

DR. MOSES

The sutures are easy to place in this proximal area if you place them first.

Dr. Stahl

Whether the fascia is cut or not, it is important to place the sutures along the horizontal axis of the flap. In this way they will interfere with the blood supply the least.

Dr. Grotting

In the case discussed in the text, Dr. Zubowicz, you were responsible for the development of a seroma in the donor area that could have been avoided had you handled the drains as I recommend. The elevation of the flap interrupts lymphatic channels in the leg. It is good practice to leave the drains in for a very long time to diminish the likelihood of seromas developing and forming mature cavities.

Dr. Zubowicz

Are there any reconstructions that you have seen or read about that just should not be done?

Dr. McKinnon

In those cases where the abdominal wall defect is unilateral, that is, eccentric and not involving both rectus columns, consider this option. The opposite-side posterior rectus fascia may be turned over to introduce a breadth of fascia equal to the width of the rectus sheath. In my experience, the blood supply to this fascia is not axial but survives. If this is adequate to close the fascial hole, you are left only with a skin-reconstruction problem.

However, conditions where a rectus turnover or turnunder flap will suffice are uncommon. My personal experience with these flaps has not been good.

Dr. Moses

As was outlined in the text, placing skin grafts on granulation tissue over mesh is a short-term solution with tremendous long-term problems. I would not recommend that.

Dr. Grotting

Another trap is the flap from one leg that just fails at the tip followed by the same flap from the opposite leg. Generally, the tip of that flap is lost as well. If it defeats you the first time, it likely will defeat you again.

DR. STAHL

I strongly agree with avoiding a skin graft over mesh. Furthermore, in cases where there has been infection, I will remove the mesh during the first hospitalization and replace it with a skin graft. Usually, the mesh is already working itself loose and is easy to remove. By this time the granulation tissue has cemented the bowel in the abdomen and the mesh is not needed to keep the viscera within the abdomen. A skin graft is easily accepted and the abdominal contents are well secured.

References

1. Dibbell DG, Mixter RC, Dibbell DG. Abdominal wall reconstruction (the "mutton chop flap"). Plast Reconstr Surg 1991;87:60–65.

2. Brown DM, Sicard GA, Flye MW, Khouri RK. Closure of complex abdominal wall defects with bilateral rectus femoris flaps with fascial extensions. Surgery 1993;114:112–116.

3. Caffee HH. Reconstruction of the abdominal wall by variations of the tensor fasciae latae flap. Plast Reconstr Surg 1983;71:348–353.

4. Peled I, Daplan H, Herson M, Wexler MR. Tensor fasciae latae musculocutaneous flap for abdominal wall reconstruction. Ann Plast Surg 1983;11:141–143.

5. Neven P, Shepherd JH, Tham KF, Fisher C, Breach N. Reconstruction of the abdominal wall with a latissimus dorsi musculocutaneous flap. Gynecol Oncol 1993;49:403–406.

6. Mathes S, Nahai F. Clinical applications of muscle and musculocutaneous flaps. St. Louis: C.V. Mosby, 1982.

7. Voles CR, Richardson JD, Bland KI, Tobin GR, Flint LM, Polk HC. Emergency abdominal wall reconstruction with polypropylene mesh. Ann Surg 1981;194:219–223.

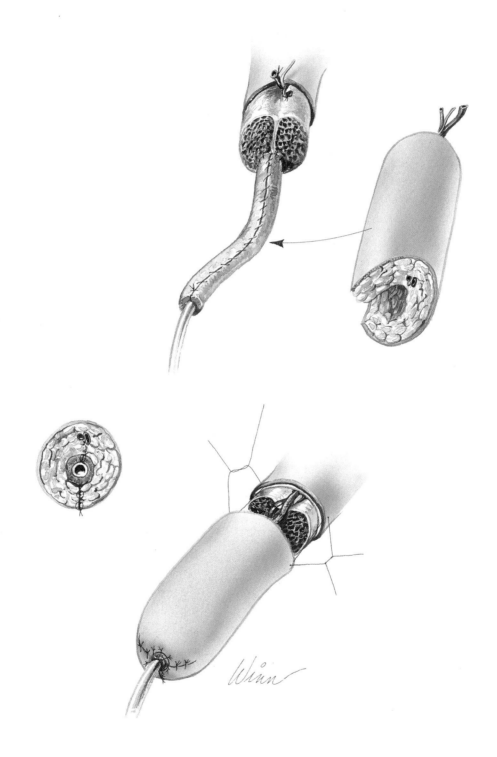

10

RECONSTRUCTION OF THE PENIS

VINCENT N. ZUBOWICZ

THE PROBLEM

A 15-year-old boy was involved in a motor vehicle accident which threw him from the car. The car partially rolled onto the victim, bringing the hot muffler to rest against the waist and thighs of the young man. As a result, the patient suffered full-thickness burns to the genital region, abdomen, and anterior thighs. There were no significant visceral or bony injuries.

It was found after several days of wound toilet that the glans, one complete corpus cavernosum, about half of the other corpus cavernosum, the entire corpus spongiosum, all the penile skin, and about half of the scrotum were totally lost. The urethra was completely destroyed to the base of the penis. Thus, only a portion of one corpus cavernosum remained of the entire penis.

INTRODUCTION

The penis serves as a urinary conduit from the bladder as well as an organ of sexual function. In this latter capacity, the penis should have erectile capability, allowing for the transmission of ejaculate, and ideally, the organ should have sensibility. Reconstruction should be aimed at satisfying these goals. Body image may be closely tied to the appearance of this sexual organ and therefore the aesthetic result is of more than passing interest.

The scrotum houses the testicles and adjusts their relationship to the coelomic cavity to maintain a temperature best suited for spermatogenesis. The scrotum must be large enough to allow independent movement of the testicles but not so large so as to rub against the inside of the thighs.

The operating microscope allows importation of blocks of tissue for penile reconstruction that can provide adequate skin for coverage of the erectile bodies, the potential for sensibility, and serve as a secondary reservoir of tissue for urethral reconstruction. There is no local tissue transfer that matches this. If suitable tissue for reconstruction exists in a donor region and there are usable arteries, veins, and nerves in the perineal region, then reconstruction by free tissue transfer is by far the procedure of choice.

PATIENT MANAGEMENT

Initial management specific to the genital burns was directed at preserving as much native tissue as possible. Conservative debridement and frequent dressing changes with physiologic solutions were employed. After stabilization of the wound (which resulted in only a portion of one erectile body remaining), reconstruction was staged in the following manner (Figure 10.1a,b).

A radial forearm flap with a branch of the cutaneous radial nerve was harvested and transferred to reconstruct the covering for the penis. The dorsal neurovascular bundle was chosen as the donor vessels and nerves. Urine was diverted by perineal urethrostomy in the wake of a suprapubic tube placed at the time of the original injury. This innervated skin unit was placed to cover the remaining corpora.

Approximately 6 weeks later, reconstruction of the urethra was performed by harvesting a patch of bladder mucosa through a suprapubic, ex-

Figure 10.1. (a, b). (a) Denuded shaft of penis covered with split-thickness skin graft. (b) Illustration of split-thickness skin graft covering shaft of penis.

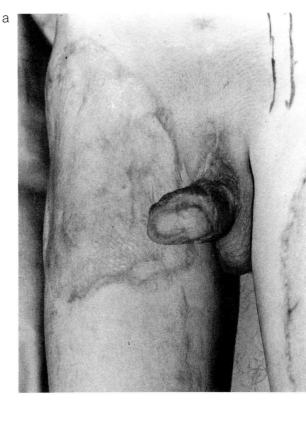

a

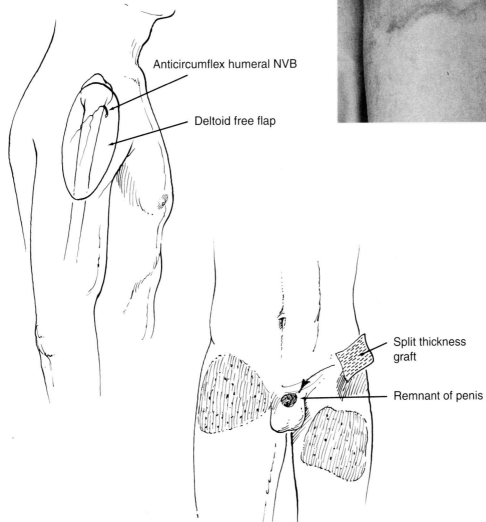

b

Anticircumflex humeral NVB

Deltoid free flap

Split thickness graft

Remnant of penis

traperitoneal approach. This rectangle of bladder was tubed with a running 6-0 plain suture and connected to the end of the native urethra. The mucosa was placed in a richly vascularized bed by tunneling it through the healthy radial forearm reconstruction on the ventral aspect (color plate on page 190).

The end of the mucosa graft was spatulated and sutured through an opening in the distal end of the radial forearm flap. A Foley catheter was placed through the mucosa graft into the bladder. The perineal urethrostomy was eliminated. The postoperative course was complicated by a slight urethral stricture at the proximal anastomosis. This was easily corrected by dilation in the office performed monthly for about 6 months.

The patient has erectile function without significant chordee. He states that there is sensibility in the flap and has successfully completed intercourse. Urination is presently normal. The patient now requests greater length and caliber of the penis. The skin is adequate to accommodate a penile prosthesis. However, the urologist will delay placement of a prosthesis until the patient is completely sexually mature (Figure 10.2a,b).

ANATOMY

The anatomy of the penis and perineum is complex. For the purposes of reconstruction, the anatomy can be simplified, considering only those layers and structures addressed during reconstructive surgery.

The skin covering of the shaft is loose and expansile, and is attached to the deeper structures by a loose adventitial layer. Sensibility to this layer is through dorsal cutaneous branches of the internal pudendal nerve. These branches are used when innervated free tissue transfers are utilized for reconstruction. The blood supply to the skin and the venous drainage are primarily on the dorsal surface, accompanying the dorsal sensory nerves. The deep inferior epigastric vessels or the femoral vessels may be used for vascular reconstitution, depending on the condition of the tissues and the character of the vessels.

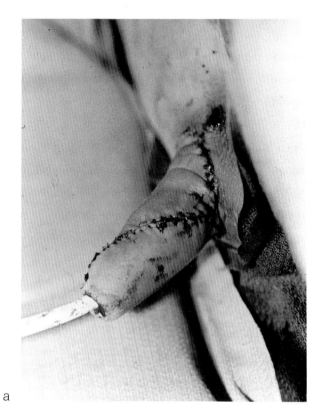

a

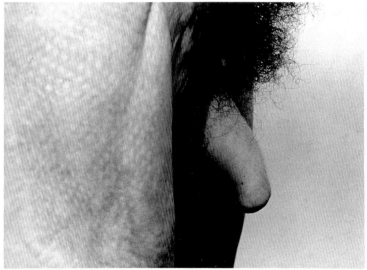

b

Figure 10.2. (a,b).   (a) Reconstruction of penis with radial forearm flap—immediate results.
(b) Reconstruction of penis after 6 months—functional as a urethral conduit and for intercourse.

The radial forearm flap is harvested from the nondominant forearm. The flap is a well-vascularized fasciocutaneous unit with blood supply delivered by perforators from the radial artery and venous drainage through the cephalic vein or concomitant veins accompanying the radial artery. The flap is designed based on measurements taken from the perineal area. The circumference is provided by the horizontal width of the flap. The length is taken from the longitudinal length and may be 10 to 12 cm depending upon the size of the forearm.

The flap affords reconstructive options after it has been raised but still attached to the native blood supply. A portion of the width, usually on the ulnar border, can be tubed into a urethra. Manipulation of the distal skin can create a hood that mimics a glans. Consideration must be given to the amount of hair growth on the forearm.

The medial and lateral antebrachial nerves traverse the area included in the flap development and are used as a cutaneous nerve supply to restore sensibility to the reconstructed penis. They are mobilized as far proximal as is practicable to allow for tension-free anastomosis to a branch of the pudendal nerve. Nerve grafts are not necessary.

DISCUSSION

As stated, the penis has two functions: as a conduit of urine and as an organ of sexual function. Neither function is a requirement for life, but in anyone who is not completely debilitated, they must be considered extremely important. It is possible to reconstruct so as to segregate function. That is, one can reconstruct a penis that functions as a urinary conduit but not as a sexual organ or the converse. Presently, with the available modern techniques, reconstruction for one function and not the other should rarely be necessary.

Local flaps can be used but will lack innervation. Groin flaps, rectus myocutaneous flaps and various thigh flaps have been described.[1-3] Most can provide tissue to mimic a penis but lack the overall versatility of free tissue transfer.

Several donor choices have been described for free tissue transfer.[4-8] Most of these provide skin, subcutaneous tissue, and innervation. The radial and ulnar free flaps have even been designed to carry a vascularized segment of bone to create rigidity.[5] Technical ease is a matter of personal opinion, as is the magnitude of donor morbidity (Figure 10.3a,b).

My own preference is for the radial forearm flap. The blood supply is predictable, as are the cutaneous sensory nerves needed for sensibility restoration. There has been, in my experience, an abundance of skin to accommodate the erectile bodies or a prosthesis if required.

The major disadvantage remains donor morbidity. A skin graft is used to cover the donor area of the forearm, and a portion of the dorsum of the hand is rendered insensate when the cutaneous nerves are harvested with the flap. The aesthetic consequences can be diminished if the patient is willing to undergo secondary reconstruction of the forearm.

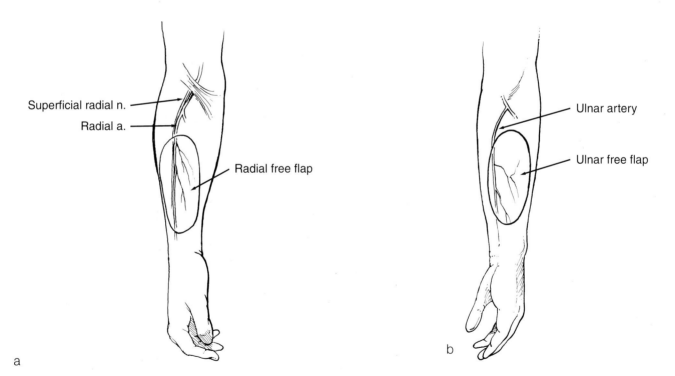

Superficial radial n.

Radial a.

Radial free flap

Ulnar artery

Ulnar free flap

a

b

Figure 10.3. (a,b).   Two vascularized skin flap options available for reconstruction of the penis.

Reconstruction of the urethra is commonly problematic. Fistulae and strictures are common.[9] Tubed skin grafts and mucosa grafts (placed, of course, in a well-vascularized bed) work well if one is willing to endure temporary urine leaks and dilate the urethra periodically. Tubed bladder mucosa placed as a free graft works exceptionally well in my experience. It is easy to harvest, although a cystotomy is necessary, and has the theoretical advantage of matching the native urethra with histologically similar tissue. The graft can be placed at the time of free tissue transfer. However, this introduces a number of variables into the reconstruction, requiring particular attention to suture lines and tissue orientation that may be unnecessary if the procedure is staged. Furthermore, any difficulties with the free tissue transfer would introduce immediate problems to the urethral reconstruction.

Bladder mucosa obviates problems of epidermal desquamation and hair growth within the urethra seen with skin grafts and skin flaps. These are not critical problems but are nuisances that can be avoided if bladder mucosa is used.

Flaps of vascularized tissue for urethral reconstruction have been fashioned from the flaps used in reconstruction.[4,6,9] There exist, however, technical difficulties with the proximal suture of reconstructed conduit to urethra as well as distal meatoplasty. Furthermore, hair growth and desquamation of keratinized epithelium may create hygiene problems. When a urethral tube is to be fashioned from the free tissue transfer, a non-hair-bearing surface should be chosen (Figure 10.4).[6]

Erectile function is obviously preserved if the corpora are intact. Skin covering may be accomplished with a simple skin graft if the corpora (including the corpus spongiosum) are present. This may not be ideal, but is at least temporarily satisfactory.[10]

Reconstruction of erectile bodies remains an unsolved problem. If the two erectile bodies are totally absent, then bulk must be provided to fill out a penis of suitable caliber for sexual function. There is no satisfactory way to reconstruct an erectile body that can change caliber on demand.

Therefore, two approaches are available. Native tissue can be used to

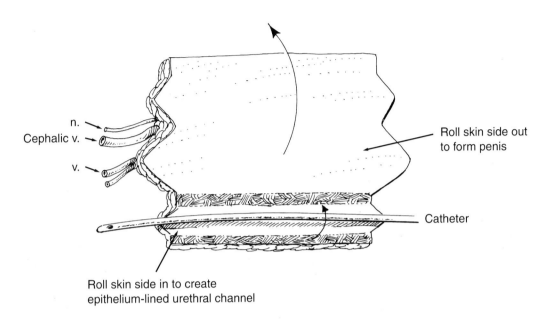

n.
Cephalic v.

v.

Roll skin side out
to form penis

Catheter

Roll skin side in to create
epithelium-lined urethral channel

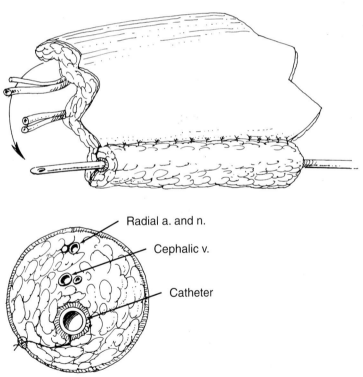

Radial a. and n.

Cephalic v.

Catheter

Figure 10.4. Illustration of one-stage reconstruction of the penis using primary urethral reconstruction from radial forearm free flap.

provide bulk. Fat or muscle is available as part of the free flap reconstruction or as local flaps. Both are static in volume and not especially rigid. The free deltoid flap, for example, may provide enough volume for even the erect penis, but a "stiffener" is required for acceptable sexual function.[6] Rib cartilage as a free graft and vascularized bone as part of a free tissue transfer create a permanently rigid shaft.[5,6,8]

Penile prostheses are available. These are composed of silicone and can be of fixed or variable volume.[9] They can be quite rigid, which is advantageous during intercourse. Prostheses are, of course, foreign bodies. They will provoke at least a mild inflammatory response. Infection and extrusion are problems that are occasionally encountered.

The glans is highly vascular and innervated. It also has rather remarkable regenerative capability after injury. Management should be most conservative until it is irrefutable that this structure has been lost. Reconstruction is aesthetic only. The characteristic shape can be approached by adjusting the distal tissues of the free tissue transfer. Micropigmentation can further highlight the differences between the glans and the shaft.

ROUNDTABLE DISCUSSION

DR. ZUBOWICZ

This patient demonstrates the problem of near-total penile reconstruction. He had the advantage of preservation of one erectile body. The corpus spongiosum and urethra were lost as a result of the accident.

The urethra required reconstruction, bladder mucosa being chosen over a split-thickness skin graft, a full-thickness skin graft, or a tubed vascularized flap. The bladder mucosa was the urologist's choice because of its similarity to urethral mucosa. Hygiene problems arising from skin grafts and tubed flaps (developed from the radial forearm flap) were thus avoided.

The radial forearm flap was chosen for covering because of its caliber, texture, and ability to be transferred as an innervated flap.

I do not see any practical role for the various local transfers, although I have used them myself. These flaps are improperly oriented, commonly too thick, and never innervated. Their only advantage is more acceptable donor morbidity compared to the various free tissue transfers available from the upper extremity.

DR. GROTTING

The plan in this case was well thought out and executed. In the past 10 years the radial forearm flap has emerged as the best available donor site for this difficult reconstruction. I prefer to perform total penile reconstruction in one stage. My preference for urethral reconstruction is to tube a segment of the radial forearm skin, creating a tube within a tube. This allows reconstruction of the phallus and urethra in one operation.

Innervation of the free tissue transfer, as was done here, is very important. Sensation provided by the dorsal sensory nerve of the penis is ideal. If these nerves have been destroyed or cannot be located, one has to dissect out the sensory branches of the pudendal nerve deeper in the groin crease.

I have approached restoration of erectile function by the insertion of rib cartilage. Anchoring of the cartilage is difficult and not commonly attempted. Nevertheless, the graft seems to undergo little if any resorption and aids in sexual function. It has the disadvantage of being permanently stiff.

One notable case illustrative of the problems of an unfixed cartilage graft occurred not long ago in one of my patients. The weight of the unsupported cartilage stretched out the skin of the reconstruction, making it extraordinarily long and very thin—abut the size of a pencil. The pressure of the cartilage in patients who have undergone reconstruction is important, however, since pressure of the cartilage (or prosthesis) on the remnant of the corporal body is important for orgasm.

Reconstructions should be broken down, as you did, into the anatomic and physiological needs of the patient. Paradoxically, partial reconstructions are often more difficult than total reconstructions. This is because the reconstruction must be tailored to include any functional anatomic remnants.

DR. ZUBOWICZ

I think the utility of innervating free tissue transfers in many circumstances is overstated in our literature. With this type of reconstruction, however, I think that it is extremely important. Sensibility contributes mightily to sexual function and satisfaction.

I can't say that I see cartilage as a real asset in embellishment of volume and length. Does it warp? Does it resorb? How often does it need to be redone?

DR. GROTTING

A certain amount of absorption takes place, but, remarkably, the bulk of the cartilage maintains its volume and does not atrophy. It probably becomes revascularized. As a matter of fact, there have been cases where we have gone back to replace cartilage that had fractured and found it to be well vascularized.

In one unusual case, we replaced a broken cartilage graft (well-vascularized, of course) with two new silicone prostheses positioned side by side. This implant functioned well without extrusion or exposure.

DR. ZUBOWICZ

Does anyone else have experience with a prosthesis to enhance volume or rigidity?

DR. MOSES

I am of the opinion that a prosthesis, any prosthesis, is more likely to extrude if it is present before sensation has returned. Extrusion is less likely after sensation has returned.

On the other hand, an unsupported skin tube will invariably shrink, exactly like a nasal reconstruction. For this reason I favor immediate placement of a bone or cartilage frame that can at least serve as a spacer, accepting the increased risk of extrusion. When sensation returns, the graft can be replaced with a better prosthesis if this is judged to be advantageous for the patient. This "spacer" graft has the additional advantage of inducing a capsule that provides further stabilization. In my experience, sensation, when it returns, is remarkably good.

DR. TOTH

In my experience, it is more difficult to reconstruct a partial amputation than to start from scratch and build an entirely new penis. However, if tissue is to be discarded before complete reconstruction, this should not include any erectile tissue.

My experience is limited to the radial forearm flap, using a "jelly-roll" modification to reconstruct the urethra simultaneously from the free tissue transfer. It is important to divert the urine stream for a period of time. Furthermore, nearly all urethrae constrict and need to be dilated after reconstruction, even if one spatulates the meatus as well as the proximal urethral anastomosis. Most strictures occur at this proximal anastomosis. I perform this operation with the urologist, who manages the perineal urethrostomy and reinstitution of urine flow.

In cases where the erectile bodies and urethra are intact but the skin has been lost on the penile shaft, skin grafts are perfectly satisfactory in providing coverage. They have, of course, the disadvantage of not being innervated. Would anyone do more than a skin graft in cases where the erectile bodies and urethra are intact?

DR. STAHL

Skin grafts, particularly in burns, demonstrate well the good results that can be obtained over the scrotum and penis (Figure 10.5). I would, however, be inclined to use a full-thickness graft over the penile shaft if I felt the shaft would accept it. Nevertheless, skin grafts, full or split thickness, are acceptable. Nothing else need be done.

DR. FRENCH

Full-thickness grafts are really never necessary. A split-thickness graft taken with a Padgett dermatome 0.16 thousandths of an inch in thickness or more works perfectly well.

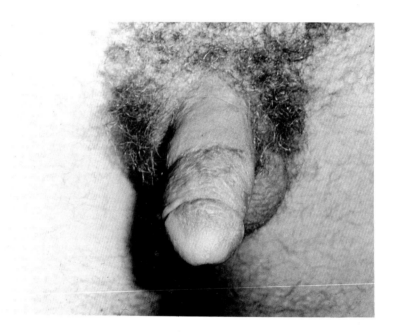

Figure 10.5. Penile shaft covered with split-thickness skin graft.

DR. ZUBOWICZ

In general, I agree, particularly when dealing with initial wound coverage. Certainly, the skin graft will accomplish a closed wound and in most circumstances be functionally adequate. However, I have had several cases, one recently, where functional disturbance to erection was observed because of a skin graft. In these cases, the skin graft was replaced electively with a vascularized and innervated free tissue transfer. The replacement allowed for more erectile length, alleviated pain associated with erection, presumably resulting from the surface restrictions of the split-thickness graft, and ultimately became innervated, which enhanced sexual function.

DR. ELLIOTT

In situations where an open wound exists, a split-thickness skin graft should be considered the favored method of coverage. The graft allows stabilization of the wound and assessment for a more sophisticated reconstruction. A skin graft may present, as has been said, long-term problems, since it is not innervated and is restrictive in terms of surface area. It can be replaced electively with a free flap such as the SIEA free flap.

Dr. Zubowicz

All of the reconstructions we have heretofore discussed yield a phallus that looks uncircumcised. Does anyone have thoughts on reconstructing the equivalent of a glans?

Dr. McKinnon

It is certainly possible to create a phallus with a glans. One technique is the use of a turnover flap. Another is deepithelializing a portion of the distal tube and turning it back on itself (Figure 10.6). However, these maneuvers introduce additional risks which must be carefully weighed against the benefits. Those benefits are aesthetic only.

Dr. French

Although it is clever to fashion a glans as part of the primary reconstruction, the primary objective is to deliver a volume of tissue that provides adequate shaft size and a urethra. This must be guaranteed first. The aesthetic reconstruction of a glans is secondary.

Dr. McKinnon

With regard to scrotal reconstruction, is it not possible or even practical to use a portion of the free tissue transfer for coverage? The radial forearm flap could be developed with a proximal extension that could be shaped to reconstruct the scrotum.

Dr. Zubowicz

I would not use an extension of a radial forearm flap to build a scrotum. In my estimation, acquiring enough surface area for total reconstruction for both penis and scrotum would be impossible. Partial reconstruction seems silly, particularly when skin grafts work so well.

I have used the SCIA (groin flap) to reconstruct the scrotum independently of penile reconstruction (Figure 10.7). Although this is a more interesting reconstruction than a skin graft, I doubt that there is any great long-term advantage. I would use such a flap only when a skin graft is technically not possible.

Dr. Toth

The shaft of the penis and the scrotum are two distinct aesthetic elements. An extension of the radial forearm flap to reconstruct the scrotum will de-

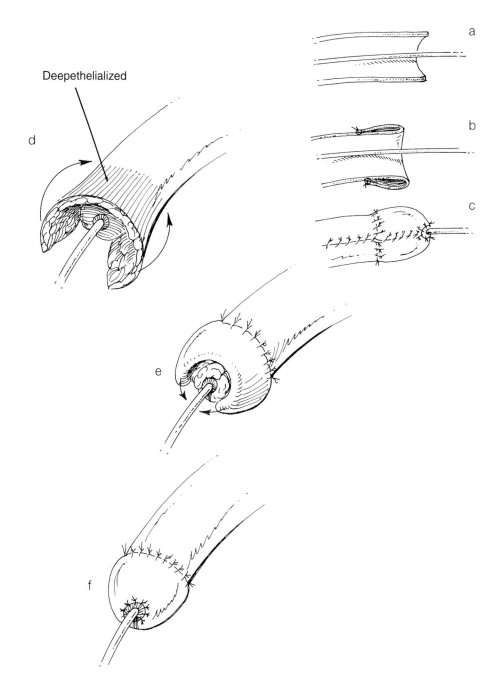

Figure 10.6. Deepithelializing a portion of the distal tube and turning it back on itself.

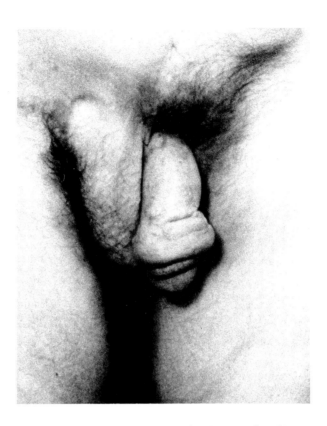

Figure 10.7. Reconstruction of the scrotum with a superficial circumflex iliac pedicle flap.

stroy the natural transition from one aesthetic unit to the other. This is yet another reason not to cover the penis and scrotum with one flap.

DR. ELLIOTT

The donor defect on the forearm, especially when such a large flap is harvested as in this case study, is certainly a problem to consider. I can think of no better alternative than the radial forearm flap for penile reconstruction, but I would prefer a flap with less donor morbidity.

In this study, expanders were used to eliminate the split-thickness graft as skin coverage for the forearm. What are the problems encountered with this type of secondary reconstruction?

DR. ZUBOWICZ

Let me respond to both your points, Dr. Elliott. I agree completely that the donor morbidity is considerable and one must carefully consider the trade-off where skin coverage has already been provided by a skin graft. Furthermore, I can think of no other flap that gives comparable advantages to the radial forearm flap, although the lateral arm flap comes close. Its donor morbidity rivals that of the radial forearm flap. The same can be said of the deltoid flap.

Reconstruction of the donor defect with skin expansion was not particularly difficult. There were no problems during the expansion and only minor wound-healing problems after final advancement of the expanded flaps and closure. Nevertheless, this is time-consuming and expensive.

DR. GROTTING

Total reconstruction of the donor defect is usually not possible. It is possible, as I have seen, to pull the expanded skin too tight and create a compressive neuropathy—to the median nerve in the case I refer to.

DR. FRENCH

The donor morbidity of the lateral arm flap is greater than that of the radial forearm flap.

DR. MOSES

The radial forearm flap is capable of carrying with it a segment of vascularized bone (radius). Is there any application of vascularized radius in structural support of the penis after reconstruction?

DR. ZUBOWICZ

I can see no applicability whatsoever, Dr. Moses, but I'm sure that you can. Would you really consider such a transfer?

DR. MOSES

Although vascularized bone is technically feasible, I think there are better ways to provide rigidity and length. Furthermore, I have never done such an operation. I would also be worried about additional donor morbidity, since I have seen plenty of cases where a portion of the radius has been harvested as part of a reconstruction and the patient has ended up with a forearm fracture.

DR. TOTH

In total penile reconstruction, augmentation of volume with cartilage or prosthetic material should be delayed. In spite of some anticipated contraction of the skin tube, the presence of a large rigid body in the tube introduces unnecessary jeopardy to the urethral anastomosis and to the integrity of the transferred tissue. Free-floating bones do not do well either.

DR. GROTTING

This idea should be biologically headed off at the pass. Bone not connected to bone will eventually disappear, resulting in costs too great to pay at both ends.

DR. ZUBOWICZ

It seems that the radial forearm flap gets the nod for reconstruction of an innervated cover in penile reconstruction. In those cases, however, where the erectile bodies are absent, what can be used to fill this innervated tube? We have heard of cartilage and possibly vascularized bone. What's wrong with a tube of muscle, such as pedicled rectus muscle? Although it would not be completely rigid, over time fibrosis would render enough stiffness to satisfy sexual needs.

DR. GROTTING

I don't believe that would work. I have had some experience with the rectus wrapping the urethra in order to prevent fistula after repair. Based on my observations in this circumstance, it is unlikely that enough rigidity would result to meet the needs of sexual function.

I am intrigued by the use of bladder mucosa for urethral reconstruction, as was done in the case study. Rather than using the mucosa as a free graft, could you not have tubed some of the bladder wall with mucosa, creating a vascularized graft that could be used for immediate urethral reconstruction?

DR. ZUBOWICZ

This was mentioned as a possibility by our urologist. The rich vascular bed achieved in this reconstruction allowed the technically simpler reconstruction by free graft. I would guess that a vascularized tube would be a definite consideration in any case where a less than optimal bed existed for a free graft.

REFERENCES

1. Song R. Total reconstruction of the male genitalia. Clin Plast Surg 1982;9:97.

2. Lai CS, Chou CK, Yang CC, Lin SD. Immediate reconstruction of the penis with an iliac flap. Br J Plast Surg 1990;43:621.

3. He Q, Lin Z, Liu Q, et al. One-stage penis reconstruction with the abdominal fasciocutaneous flap based on the double arteries. Chin Med J 1987;100:255.

4. Mackay DR, Pottie R, Kadwa MA, Stott RSH. Reconstruction of the penis using a radial forearm free flap. SAMJ 1989;76:278.

5. Koshima I, Tai T, Yamasaki M. One-stage reconstruction of the penis using an innervated radial forearm osteocutaneous flap. J Reconstr Microsurg 1986;3:19.

6. Harashina T, Inoue T, Tanaka I, Imai K, Hatoko M. Reconstruction of penis with free deltoid flap. Br J Plast Surg 1990;43:217.

7. Upton J, Mutimer KL, Loughlin K, Ritchie J. Penile reconstruction using the lateral arm flap. J R Coll Surg Edinb 1987;32:97.

8. Glasson DW, Lovie MJ, Duncan GM. The ulnar forearm free flap in penile reconstruction. Aust NZ J Surg 1986;56:477.

9. Jordan GH, Gilbert DA, Devine CJ. Male external genital reconstruction. AUA Update Series 1992;XI(27).

10. Vincent MP, Horton CE, Devine CJ. An evaluation of skin grafts for reconstruction of the penis and scrotum. Clin Plast Surg 1982;15:

6

DECISION MAKING IN PERINEAL RECONSTRUCTION

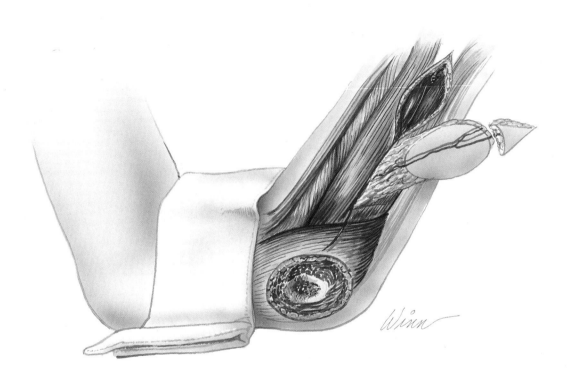

Ischial Pressure Sore Reconstruction with V-Y Hamstring Advancement Flap Reconstruction

RICHARD S. STAHL

The Problem

A 20-year-old college freshman was referred for a nonhealing ischial pressure sore. She had been paraplegic since childhood as a result of resection of a histologically benign spinal cord tumor. She had never previously suffered from pressure ulceration.

Examination demonstrated a pressure sore whose cutaneous orifice measured 3 cm (Figure 11.1a-b). The cutaneous margins were undermined for 4 cm; ischial bone was exposed at the base. Superficial necrotic tissue and exudate were present within the wound.

After an interval of preparatory wound care, improved nutrition, and counseling about pressure sore prevention, the patient was taken to the operating room for resection of the pressure sore and flap reconstruction. A "V-Y" hamstring advancement flap was chosen to satisfy the resectional defect (Figure 11.1c-f).

She was managed on a flotation bed postoperatively. Uneventful healing followed, and the patient was gradually mobilized.

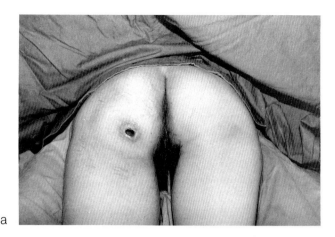

a

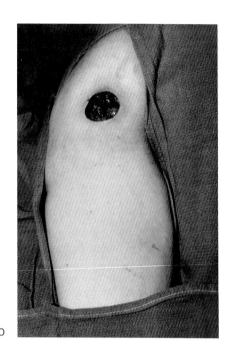

b

Figure 11.1. (a, b).   (a) Left ischial pressure sore is seen with patient in prone jackknife position. When wound closure is performed with the patient in this position, it is easily confirmed that the closure will later tolerate the sitting position without undue tension. Upon probing the wound, it is evident that there is significant undermining. Adequate debridement or resection of the wound usually results in a wound that is significantly larger than is evident externally. (b) The wound is seen after resection. As expected, the wound in need of coverage is larger than its external appearance would imply. The resection included all abnormal skin and subcutaneous tissues, the pseudobursa lining the cavity, and the ischial bony prominence.

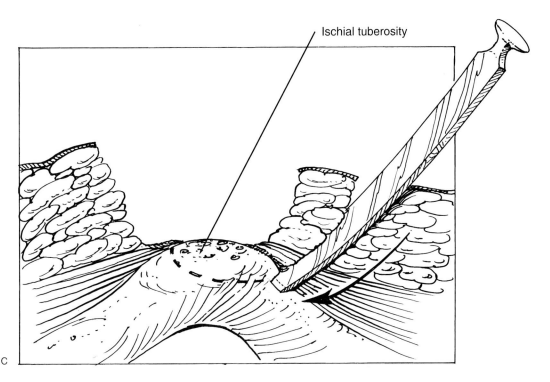

Ischial tuberosity

c

Figure 11.1. (c, d).   (c) The line drawing depicts *in continuity*
excision of the pseudobursa and ischial ostectomy. (d) After wound
resection and jet lavage, a long, wide, "V-Y" partial hamstring flap is
elevated. Tension-free inset was achieved, suturing the hamstring
origins to the gluteus and periosteal tissues superiorly, with 2-0
absorbable sutures. The donor and recipient sites were well drained
with closed-suction catheters.

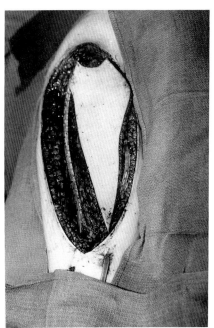

d

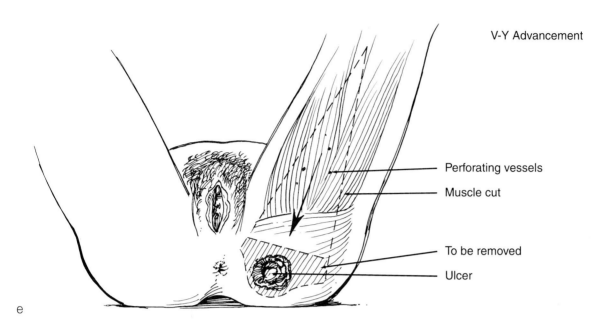

V-Y Advancement

Perforating vessels

Muscle cut

To be removed

Ulcer

e

Figure 11.1. (e, f, g). (e) Line drawing depicts area of resection (shaded) and planned flap advancement. (f) Appearance of wound at completion of closure. (g) The healed wound is seen 6 months later.

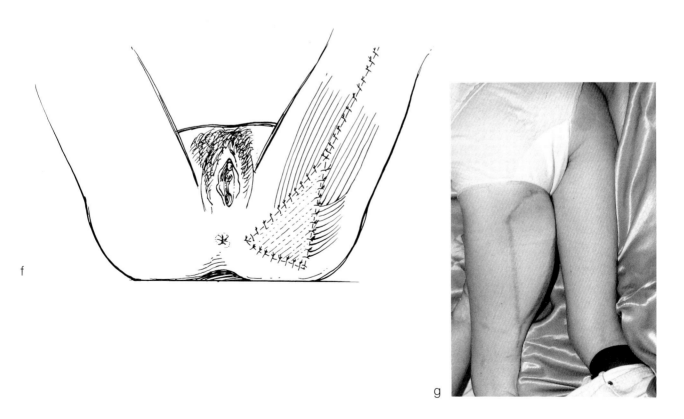

f

g

Treatment of recurrent pressure sore with re-advancement of a V-Y hamstring flap is seen in Figure 11.2.

INTRODUCTION

No more vexing and difficult a body region exists for the surgeon—especially the reconstructive surgeon—than the perineum. In this region a host of considerations impede successful surgery.

The perineum is the site of origin of the lower extremities, with their complex neurovascular an musculoskeletal components, and orifices of the alimentary and genitourinary tracts. Unlike the upper trunk, this region has weight-bearing responsibilities during sitting and standing. Accordingly, the lower extremities are dependent and adjacent to one another instead of being laterally apposed, as are the upper extremities.

The junctions of the perineum with the lower extremities form a unique, concave, cleftlike median raphe. Hidden in this midline cleft are the anus and genitourinary structures, with their specialized functions and vulnerabilities.

These invaginated contours, the multiple anatomic fusion planes and tissue types, the remoteness of the region from the individual's examining senses, and a psychosocial overlay of modesty, make diagnosis, primary treatment, surgical reconstruction, and wound care and hygiene more challenging and difficult than for any other region in the body.

AVAILABLE RECONSTRUCTIVE UNITS

There is an abundant selection of flaps available for use in perineal applications (Tables 11.1 and 11.2). These reconstructive units are found in the thigh, the buttock, the abdominal wall, and the peritoneum. Factors such as arc of rotation, degree of contamination, potential donor morbidity, and the location and type of previous surgical and radiotherapeutic interventions relative to the flap and its pedicle all have an influence on the flap choice in reconstruction.

In the perineum, especially, effective planning must also include

TABLE 11.1   INDICATIONS FOR PERINEAL RECONSTRUCTION.

Congenital	*Acquired*
Vaginal aplasia	Pressure sore
Imperforate anus	Trauma
Rectovaginal fistula	Tumor ablation
	Radiation therapy
	Postsurgical complications
	Infection

TABLE 11.2   AVAILABLE RECONSTRUCTIVE UNITS.

Gracilis	Fasciocutaneous
Gluteus	Medial thigh
Gluteal thigh	Pudendal
Tensor fascia-lata	Labial
Rectus abdominis	Perineal
Omentum	Rectus femoris
Mesentery	Sartorius

factors relating to the etiology of the wound and prognosis for recovery, concurrent procedures, requirements for positioning, three-dimensional contours affecting arcs of rotation and tunnel location during and after the operation, adequacy of exposure for safe debridement and innermost flap inset, and provisions for function of multiple regional organ systems.

SELECTED FLAP: "V-Y" HAMSTRING ADVANCEMENT

Of the many utilitarian flaps available for perineal reconstruction, the "V-Y" hamstring advancement flap is selected for discussion. It allows the reconstructive surgeon to readily recruit abundant tissue from the thigh to satisfy the most common indication for perineal reconstructive surgery: pressure sore formation. Furthermore, it is well suited for treatment of all too frequent recurrent pressure ulceration with multiple readvancement (Figure 11.2), thus sparing valuable adjacent donor units for later use.

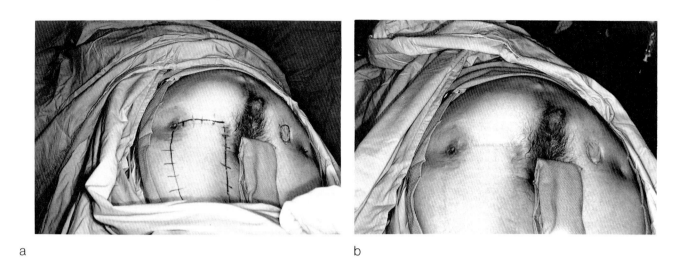

a   b

Figure 11.2. (a, b). This paraplegic patient was admitted for treatment of a left posterior trochanteric pressure sore resulting from a faulty wheelchair cushion. She had been treated for multiple bilateral pressure sores in the past. A gracilis musculocutaneous flap had been used to repair a right ischial pressure sore (see skin island). A "V-Y" hamstring musculocutaneous flap had been called upon to close a left ischial pressure sore on the left, which remained healed. A smaller, but similar, right posterior trochanteric pressure sore had been previously treated with excision and closure as well. (c) The left posterior trochanteric pressure sore was excised and closed by elevating and readvancing the previously utilized left "V-Y" hamstring flap. (d) The healed, readvanced flap is seen 9 months later. The same flap was readvanced for its third use to treat a recurrent sore 16 months postoperatively.

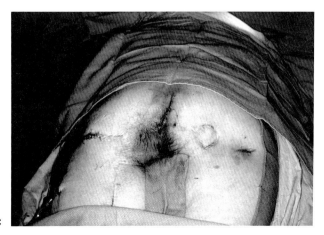

c

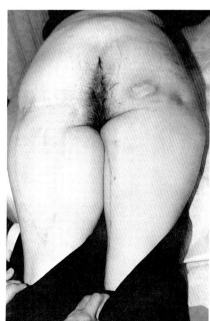

d

Anatomy

The hamstring muscles—biceps fermoris, semitendinosus, and semimembranosus—are "prime knee flexors . . . they function in normal gait to decelerate leg swing immediately prior to heel strike, thus contributing to forward momentum of the thigh and upper body."[1,2] Sacrifice of the biceps femoris muscle is well tolerated in paraplegics but may result in disability in ambulatory patients.[3]

These muscles have a common origin from the ischial tuberosity, except for the short head of the biceps femoris, which originates from the linea aspera of the femur. The biceps femoris (laterally) gradually diverges from the semimembranosus and the semitendinosus (medially) as they approach the knee, ultimately forming the lateral and medial borders of the popliteal space, respectively. The biceps inserts on the fibular head, while the semitendinosus and the semimembranosus insert onto the medial condyle of the tibia.

The sciatic nerve passes beneath the biceps femoris origin and "bisects the two hamstring muscle groups in the midline of the thigh. The common peroneal nerve passes beneath the biceps femoris tendon"[4] as it approaches the fibular head. Its motor innervation arises from the sciatic nerve. Its territory derives its sensory innervation from the posterior cutaneous nerve of the thigh.

The blood supply of this flap is segmental and arises from branches of the profunda femoris vessels. The lower third has some blood supply from popliteal branches.

Technique of Flap Elevation

The patient is placed in the prone, jackknife position to optimize exposure and accentuate the resectional defect at the recipient site, ensuring that adequate flap advancement and fill will be achieved. Prior to the initiation of the procedure, culture-specific parenteral antibiotics are administered. It is also important to have administered a bowel prep to prevent intraoperative or early postoperative soilage.

Complete resection of the pressure ulcer, with the help of methylene blue staining, must be achieved—*en bloc*, if possible—to achieve successful healing. This should include the cutaneous margins of the wound, the entire bursa-like lining that forms at pressure sore sites, and the underlying bony prominence. Once adequate resection is performed, the wound's bacterial count is further reduced with jet lavage irrigation.

A generous triangular island of skin is incised over the posterior thigh, utilizing the perforating vessels of the underlying hamstring muscles to vasculize the flap. Although it has been suggested that the superior triangular flap width be designed to correspond with the width of the resectional defect,[5] an even wider design allows for more future readvancement contingencies. Similarly, the longitudinal extent of the flap should be quite generous, comprising three-quarters to four-fifths of the length of the thigh.

The distal insertions of the hamstrings are identified inferiorly. Dissection is continued from distal to proximal along the margins of the hamstring muscles. The origins of the short and long heads of the biceps femoris are freed from the linea aspera and from beneath the gluteus maximus, respectively. If necessary to achieve adequate advancement, the hamstring insertions can be divided in the nonambulatory patient. Otherwise, they can be divided upon subsequent readvancement as needed.

Mobilization of the muscle bellies themselves is performed to increase flap advancement. During this process, perforating vessels can be variably identified and skeletonized. Once ischial origins, distal insertion, and cutaneous and muscular margins are freed, the flap is isolated solely on its vascular pedicles. Division of some distal perforators has also been described to augment flap advancement.[5]

Absorbable sutures are utilized to secure closure of the deepest layer of the wound over suction catheters. These sutures should approximate divided hamstring muscle origins to the inferior gluteal margin and/or ischial periosteum. When more vascularized fill is necessary, advancement of some inferior gluteal fibers can supplement the hamstring flap volume. It is critical to achieve closure without tension in this jackknifed position, or dehiscence will inevitably occur when the patient assumes the sitting position.

A meticulous layered closure is then performed on the cutaneous portion of the flap, actively advancing and closing the "V-Y" donor site component of the flap over suction catheters. OpSite is applied as an occlusive dressing to the entire area, securing the flap to the surrounding unoperated skin. This not only protects the fresh incisions from early soiling but mechanically "splints" the closure and minimizes distractional forces that can occur with early turning and transfers.

The patient is transferred to the Clinitron bed in the prone flat position (with the bed turned on). Turning of the patient to the supine position is then easily achieved within the bed. If general anesthesia has been employed, tracheal extubation can be safely performed. Bed rest is maintained for 2 to 3 weeks before a gradually progressive regimen of mobilization is undertaken. Participation of active and interested rehabilitation consultants is essential to make certain that appropriate padding, cushions, and wheelchairs are utilized, lest recurrent ulceration occur.

Pitfall

This flap, when elevated as described, is a hearty flap that can deliver a significant amount of tissue to the ischial area. Problems can arise, however, with intraoperative injury to the sciatic nerve. This can be problematic even in some paralyzed patients, such as those with spastic paralysis, who can experience a troublesome imbalance of spasticity.

If a large amount of tissue is required at too superior a site on the perineum, the surgeon might be tempted to mobilize the hamstring flap excessively. Overly aggressive mobilization and skeletonization of the flap can violate too many perforators and induce problems with flap ischemia.

Finally, the biceps femoris muscle should not be defunctionalized in the ambulatory patient, since it may well cause a problem with gait.

DISCUSSION

The reconstructive needs of the perineum have been shown to be demanding and variable. Indications for such interventions can include traumatic, ablative, and congenital etiologies. Wounds in this area are susceptible to mechanical stresses of lower extremity and trunk motion, maceration, and urinary and fecal contamination.

The surgeon is best prepared to meet the demands of this body region with a diverse portfolio of surgical options, flaps, techniques, and principles. He or she also must understand the three-dimensional anatomy and physiology of the region.

Each factor predisposing to poor wound healing must be addressed: contamination, devitalized tissue, radiation, glucose intolerance, steroid dependency, fistula, etc. The best and most elegant flap design and execution cannot compensate for inadequate debridement or tissue oxygenation, for example.

Many patients undergoing reconstructive surgery in this area are prone to recurrent problems in the future. Forethought must therefore also be given to long-term flap requirements and the preservation of the territories for future use. At the same time, the solution of a current problem should not be compromised by using an inadequate flap to preserve more substantial flaps for future possible problems.

Donor sites of pedicled flaps that can address perineal defects are located in the abdomen and thigh. Each reconstructive unit has its advantages and disadvantages. For example, the gracilis musculocutaneous flap can rotate anteriorly or posteriorly to satisfy defects of the groin, perineum, vagina, penis, scrotum, or anorectum. It can address an ischial pressure sore without sacrificing a flap that might later be needed for another site. It provides enough tissue bulk for only a relatively small sore, however. Furthermore, its cutaneous territory can be unreliable, especially in the obese patient or in its distal extent.

The gluteus is a source of abundant, well-vascularized, hearty tissue that can be recruited for a variety of recipient sites about the pelvis and perineum in many forms. One would not want to employ it for a small ischial wound such as that descried above, however. It would be preferable to preserve it for the more difficult sacral wound that the same patient is likely to sustain at a later time.

The gluteal thigh flap can be elevated with relative ease, with or without the gluteus maximus muscle. It can transfer a large cutaneous territory of the posterior thigh on the descending branch of the inferior gluteal artery. Such a unit can reach high into the pelvis or satisfy a large sacral or pelvic wound. Its rotation can be awkward at times, creating sizeable dog-ears in some cases. When deepithelialized, it can be used partially or wholly for vascularized fill.

The tensor fascia lata can be employed as a musculofascial or a musculofasciocutaneous flap to address defects of the groin or perineum. Perineal applications are relatively distant for this somewhat thin flap, however. It is thus unable to deliver a large amount of hearty tissue to the medial or central perineal region. The rectus femoris is more bulky than the tensor fascia lata but has a similar arc of rotation, making it an "alternative" flap[6] in many cases.

The rectus abdominis musculocutaneous flap can be an important answer to many reconstructive needs of the pelvic and perineal region. Based on the deep inferior epigastric vessels, it can support a large volume of vascularized tissue that can be transposed or tunneled subcutaneously or transperitoneally for vascularized fill or coverage or vaginal reconstruction. It requires careful attention to hernia-free closure of the abdominal donor site. Its harvest must also be carefully planned when abdominal stomas have been or will be performed concomitantly.

The greater omentum can be a valuable tool in the reconstructive surgeon's armamentarium. Unless violated by previous laparotomy, the omental flap's pedicle can be developed to achieve unsurpassed lengths. Furthermore, it can deliver a rewarding volume of extremely well-vascularized tissue to the pelvis and perineum. Finally, it can thrive in adverse conditions of contamination or radiation.

In occasional cases mesentery can be preserved as a flap when bowel resection is performed for benign disease. One or two sets of mesenteric vessels may be strategically divided, utilizing flow from more remote mesenteric vessels via arcades. In these select cases, such flap skeletonization will allow these well-vascularized tissues to be delivered to the pelvis or central perineum.

ROUNDTABLE DISCUSSION

DR. STAHL

The perineum can be a very difficult area in which to perform reconstruction. Its needs are quite varied and require a tailored, individualized plan. I think that the choice of flaps in this body region is a controversial one.

DR. ELLIOTT

My flap of choice for pressure sores is the posterior thigh flap because I feel that the skin island is very reliable. The axis of rotation is close to the ischium itself. In fact, it is proximal to the ischium, since it is the continuation of the inferior gluteal artery. You can create a fairly large flap that can be deepithelialized and can fill an undermined defect as well as provide skin coverage over it. The gracilis is a time-tested muscle or musculocutaneous flap, but the arc of rotation is 10 cm away from the ischium and the distal skin island is less than reliable, so it has drawbacks from that standpoint. The hamstring "V-Y" advancement flap is also an option for this area, but the skin closure is right on the area of maximum tension with flexion at the hip, and dehiscence can occur.

DR. ZUBOWICZ

The gracilis makes a much better free tissue transfer than it does a local flap. The bulk of the muscle is proximal where the pedicle is, and generally you use the belly of the muscle for rotation rather than as a soft tissue fill. I think the skin island is not reliable except in the thinnest of people, because in the obese person it is a gamble. My inclination would be to use the gracilis in the cases of smaller wounds because it is very much an expendable muscle.

DR. GROTTING

I agree with the traditional orientation of the skin island and with the gracilis being less than reliable distally, but most of the perforators to the skin over the gracilis come through the proximal portion. It is thus possible to outline a cutaneous island transversely oriented high in the thigh for smaller ischial defects. We have used the gracilis on many occasions for small ischial pressure sores, and particularly the ones that are quite deep. I think that the gracilis is often an ideal way to try to get muscle into the depths of the wound.

The problem with the posterior thigh flap is that although the arc of rotation is satisfactory to reach the ischium, it is a matter of rotating the flap virtually 180° in order to get to that point, and I find that in some patients it is stiff no matter how you deepithelialize the tip of the flap; it is sometimes awkward to turn that in and get good skin-to-skin closure in the ischium. One thing to keep in mind for extensive ischial pressure sores is that the descending branches of the inferior gluteal artery can sometimes be damaged, either eroded from the initial wound or damaged during the debridement.

DR. ELLIOTT

Gluteus probably should be mentioned as an island myocutaneous flap, because it provides extremely healthy muscle that can be rotated down over the ischium, as well as having a very hearty overlying skin island. I usually reserve the gluteus for the sacral area.

DR. ZUBOWICZ

I'd like to raise a question about positioning of the patient at the time of the operation. Does it make a difference to you in planning other positioning on the operating table or the ultimate execution of the flap?

DR. STAHL

One would like to simulate the most demanding position the flap will have to withstand. Thus one can ensure that enough tissue will be delivered to the wound. For example, the patient can be jackknifed in the prone position.

DR. ELLIOTT

The posterior perineum includes not only ischial problems but also those of the more central posterior perineum, such as the total colectomy wounds with radiation or vaginal reconstruction after pelvic exenteration. In addition to the flaps we talked about, the rectus abdominis myocutaneous flap can be tubed and turned down to reconstruct the vagina.

DR. ZUBOWICZ

Following up on Dr. Elliott's comment—for those cases that involve the pelvic floor as part of the perineal reconstruction, such as the abdominoperineal resection or pelvic exenteration, I agree strongly that the rectus abdominis is the ideal solution to the problem. In these circumstances, muscles from the leg are severely limited by arcs of rotation. The rectus muscle is an axial flap on its pedicle; it can be twisted, turned, and basically put in a number of positions to take care of the reconstructive needs.

DR. TOTH

Since some of these abdominoperineal wounds have associated abdominal stomas, it can be very difficult both in terms of morbidity and obtaining adequate tissue bulk. The rectus is therefore sometimes not available as an option.

DR. ZUBOWICZ

If the procedure can be planned with the surgical oncologist, the stoma is simply placed out of the way of the rectus that one chooses to use. That solves the problem. I also think it's important in those cases that you go through adequate preparation of the bowel and so forth to prevent or at least reduce the risk of morbidity from infection.

DR. ZUBOWICZ

I think that the muscles of the leg are certainly much more expendable in the paraplegic patient than the muscles in the abdomen.

DR. TOTH

I have one concern about taking the rectus abdominis in a patient who has an ostomy. In a patient in whom abdominal wall integrity is important, I have definite concerns about weakening the abdominal wall, particularly as this patient gets older. In terms of flap selection, I don't see any magic, particularly with regard to muscle, and my choice would have been the inferior gluteal thigh flap, the posterior thigh flap, in terms of being able to bring up an adequate amount of tissue.

REFERENCES

1. Tobin GR. Biceps femoris flaps. In: Strauch B, Vasconez L, Hall-Findlay E, editors. Encyclopedia of Flaps. Boston: Little, Brown and Co., 1990:1618.

2. Simon SR, Mann RA, Hagy JL, Larsen LJ. Role of the posterior calf muscles in normal gait. J Bone Joint Surg 1978;60A:469.

3. Mathes S, Nahi F. Anterior thigh. In: Clinical Atlas of Muscle and Musculocutaneous Flaps. St. Louis: C.V. Mosby Co., 1979:318–328.

4. McCraw J, Arnold PG. McCraw and Arnold's atlas of muscles and musculocutaneous flaps. Norfolk, Va.: Hampton Press, 1986:377–378.

5. Hurteau JE, Bostwick J, Nahai F, Hester R, Jurkiewicz MJ. V-Y advancement of hamstring musculocutaneous flap for coverage of ischial pressure sores. Plast Reconstr Surg 1981;68:539–542.

6. Mathes SJ, Eshima I. The principles of muscle and musculocutaneous flaps. In: McCarthy JG, editor. Plastic Surgery. Philadelphia: W.B. Saunders Co., 1990:397–399.

12

GROIN AND PERINEAL WOUNDS

JAMES H. FRENCH, JR.

THE PROBLEM

An adult paraplegic man presented with a chronic wound of the perineum and left groin. The wound had been previously debrided and was associated with osteomyelitis of the pelvis. The wound measured 7×9 cm. The superior aspect of the wound was immediately overlying and included the pelvic bone. The patient had a history of recurrent pressure sores and had multiple scars over the anterior lateral aspect of the left thigh and hip. In addition, he had old scars on his left gluteal area. The scars appeared to be associated with old rotation flaps. The problem is one of a large pressure sore of the left groin and perineum that has bony involvement.

INTRODUCTION

There are many muscles or myocutaneous flaps available for coverage of groin and perineal wounds.[3] The lower extremity and abdomen serve as the source for most of these tissues, and certainly free tissue transfer broadens our options. The posterior thigh also has the ability to donate tissues to the perineum in certain cases.

The objective in the management of this case is to cover the open wound with well-vascularized tissue that serves not only as covering but also as a combatant to previously documented osteomyelitis. Adequate debridement and intravenous antibiotics in conjunction with muscle flap coverage have been shown to be effective in the management of osteomyelitis.

The rectus abdominis muscle or myocutaneous flap based on the inferior epigastric vessels is an excellent choice for closing difficult groin and perineal wounds. There are multiple examples and case reports in the literature that support utilization of this flap for such wounds.[4,5,6]

DISCUSSION

The inferiorly based rectus abdominis muscle was the flap of choice in this case for several reasons. The size of the wound and the associated osteomyelitis required a substantial amount of muscle and/or soft tissue. The fact that the patient had numerous scars on the ipsilateral thigh and buttock from previous rotation flaps eliminated certain options.

The arc of rotation based on the inferior epigastric vessels is more than adequate to cover the groin and perineum. The extended deep inferior epigastric flap as described by Taylor et al.[1] increases that rotational arc significantly and permits coverage of more distant wounds. The skin island is utilized and oriented according to the specific needs of the wound. In this case a vertical skin island was raised in anticipation of the need for additional soft tissue bulk. The decision was later made to discard the skin island in favor of a split-thickness skin graft.

The blood supply provided by the deep inferior epigastric artery makes this an extremely reliable muscle or myocutaneous flap.[7] The cutaneous territories supplied by the periumbilical perforators allow for a wide range of design and bulk for the skin islands.[9] The size and quality of the rectus abdominis muscle obviously vary from patient to patient, but even more so in patients with neurologic deficits. Pena et al.[2] discovered the muscles to be atrophic and fibrotic in a series of eight neurologically impaired patients, even though some of the patients had T-10 and T-11 lesions. In our case the patient had a large healthy muscle with no evidence of atrophy. This was considered an advantage in covering the wound and the exposed bone. Concerns have been expressed in the literature about sacrificing the rectus abdominis muscle in a paraplegic patient. In our patient and in other reported cases, no appreciable postoperative problems arose from sacrificing the rectus abdominis muscle.

In summary, the inferiorly based rectus abdominis muscle is an excellent choice for closure of groin and perineal wounds. Its reliability is well documented and its versatility has been demonstrated throughout the literature. The ease with which the flap is raised and transferred to the area of concern is also a major advantage. Its arc of rotation and blood supply allow a significant amount of well-vascularized tissue to be transferred to the groin and perineal areas without compromise.

Technique

The patient was placed in the lithotomy position. The 7×9 cm ulceration in the left groin was excised and debrided adequately. A proposed skin island was outlined over the left periumbilical perforators and oriented in a vertical dimension (Figures 12.1 and 12.2). The skin island was incised circumferentially down to the rectus fascia. A vertical incision was made from the superior and inferior aspects of the island and again extended down to the rectus fascia. The rectus fascia was incised superiorly and inferiorly from the skin island and the muscle was separated from its medial and lateral attachments. Because of the need for a large muscle mass, the entire muscle was sacrificed. The muscle was divided with the cautery near its insertion and the superior epigastric vessels were ligated. The myocutaneous flap was raised in an inferior direction (Figure 12.3). The inferior epigastric vessels were identified and protected. A subcutaneous tunnel was created between the abdominal wound and the problem area in the left groin. The

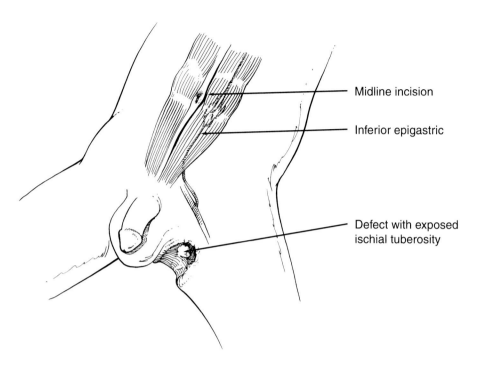

Midline incision

Inferior epigastric

Defect with exposed
ischial tuberosity

Figure 12.1. Wound and proposed rectus abdominis muscle flap.

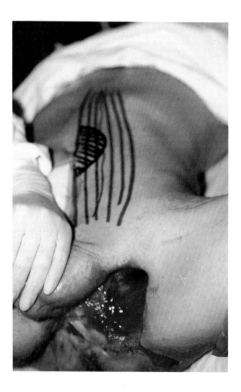

Figure 12.2. Demonstration of extent of wound.

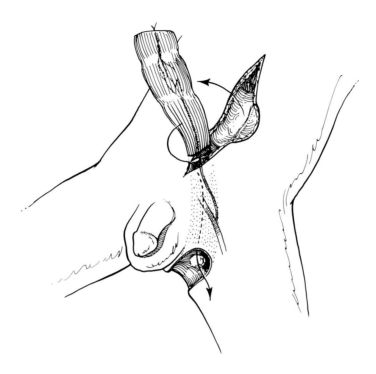

Figure 12.3. The raised myocutaneous flap.

tunnel should be of adequate size to avoid compression and vascular compromise. If more length or mobility is needed, the origin of the muscle can be divided. Care must be taken to protect the pedicle if the origin is divided. The myocutaneous flap was then pulled through the tunnel and positioned appropriately (Figures 12.4 and 12.5). If the skin island is too bulky (as in this case), it can be removed and the exposed muscle covered with a split thickness of skin graft. Suction drains were placed beneath the transposed flap and the donor site. The anterior rectus fascia was closed with a running 0 nonabsorbable suture. The remainder of the wound was closed in a standard fashion (Figures 12.6 and 12.7).

ANATOMY

The anatomy of the rectus abdominis muscle and the myocutaneous flap has been well described. The transverse rectus abdominis myocutaneous

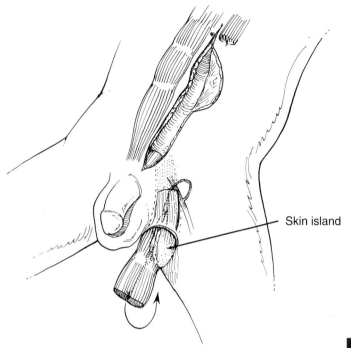

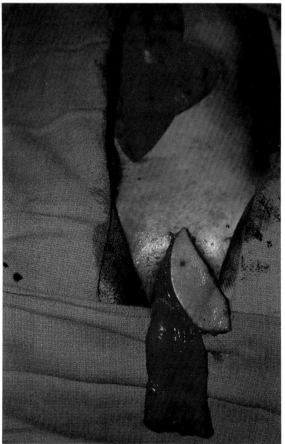

Figure 12.4. Muscle flap covering wound.

Skin island

Figure 12.5. Flap raised and tunneled through to wound.

Figure 12.6. Flap sewn in place with split-thickness skin graft coverage.

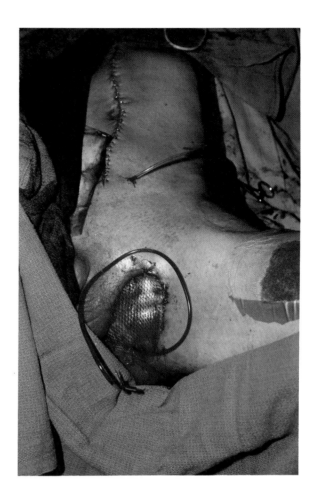

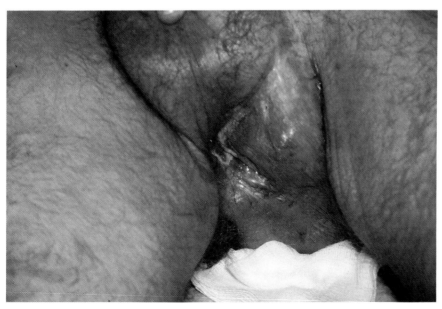

Figure 12.7. Wound several months postoperatively.

(TRAM) flap, based on the superior epigastric vessels, is the most frequently used form of breast reconstruction that uses autologous tissue. The concepts and principles involved in raising the inferiorly based flap are the same. The inferior epigastric artery enters the rectus abdominis muscle obliquely in the lower lateral aspect of the muscle. It courses along the posterior surface of the muscle and then penetrates the muscle in the vicinity of the arcuate line. The arterioles that provide the supply of the skin and subcutaneous tissue of the abdominal wall are located between the arcuate line and the costal margins, but are concentrated in the periumbilical area. In designing skin islands, these anatomic relationships must be considered. The inferiorly based flap is more reliable than the superiorly based because the inferior epigastric vessel is the dominant vessel to the level of the costal margin in the majority of patients.

The muscle inserts into the costal cartilage of the fifth, sixth, and seventh ribs, and can be divided at its insertion or more inferiorly, depending on the needs of the wound to be covered. In addition, only the central portion of the muscle need be utilized with the overlying skin island if muscle bulk is not an important component of the flap.

The inferior epigastric artery can be traced to the external iliac artery if a lengthy pedicle is needed. This maneuver is usually accompanied by the division of the muscle origin from the pubic crest and symphysis pubis.

In general, the anatomy of the rectus abdominis muscle is constant and well defined, allowing for relative ease of surgical dissection.

Roundtable Discussion

Dr. French

This is the case of a chronic paraplegic patient who had a very significant groin wound with associated osteomyelitis. The flap that was chosen was a rectus abdominis myocutaneous flap. The reason it was chosen was that I was concerned about the quality of the muscle in his lower extremities and the ability of that muscle to cover exposed bone or bone that had been involved with osteomyelitis. I raised the flap, and then after raising the flap, decided I didn't need the skin and subcutaneous tissue and I discarded it and used a split-thickness skin graft to cover the muscle. The wound healed without a problem. In this T-12 paraplegic patient, missing one rectus abdominis muscle has not represented a problem.

Dr. Zubowicz

Dr. French, I can't make a strong case against your approach to the problem, although I do think that the muscles of the leg are certainly much more expendable in the paraplegic patient than the muscles in the abdomen. For that reason I think I would have at least taken a surgical look at those muscles to see if your presumptions about whether or not they would be satisfactory for the reconstruction are valid. Other than that, I think it's an appropriately legitimate way of approaching the problem.

Dr. Elliott

I think that there are definitely other choices that are probably higher on the list for this problem, including the gracilis, which is a little smaller in bulk but is very proximate to the wound. The rectus femoris is another excellent choice. It could be rotated in, or the posterior thigh flap is a nonmuscle choice, and I'm not sure that muscle is a necessary ingredient to achieve a healed wound. I have used the rectus for the perineal problems myself, but it has always been down the line after choices have eroded through and are not available.

Dr. Grotting

I agree with the traditional orientation of the skin island and with the gracilis being less than reliable distally, but this has been studied by the Milwaukee

Group, and most of the perforators to the skin of the gracilis come through the proximal portion, and it's possible to outline a cutaneous island transversely oriented high in the thigh that can be used to advantage for smaller ischial defects. We have used the gracilis on many occasions for small ischial pressure sores, and particularly the ones that are quite deep. I think that the gracilis often is an ideal way to try to get muscle into the depths of the wound. The problem with the posterior thigh flap is that although the arc of rotation is satisfactory to reach the ischium, it's a matter of rotating the flap virtually 180° to get to that point, and I find that in some patients it is stiff no matter how you deepithelialize the tip of the flap; it's sometimes awkward to turn that in and get good skin-to-skin closure in the ischium. The use of the combination of the two flaps, when perhaps you could get by with one, can be criticized, but for larger defects I think it is sometimes a good choice. One thing to keep in mind for extensive ischial pressure sores is that the descending branches of the inferior gluteal artery sometimes can be damaged, either eroded from the initial wound or damaged during the debridement. So one shouldn't commit oneself too soon for that.

DR. MCKINNON

I think that this case well represents the notion that there are lots of ways to skin this cat. The problem of an ischial pressure sore really can be adequately taken care of with any of the flaps you mentioned. My own choice in this case might have been the gracilis, since there is such a small amount of surgery to be done and the transposition point of a vascular pedicle is so small.

DR. ZUBOWICZ

In raising a question about positioning of the patient at the time of the operation, as concerns the position of the flap with the thigh extended as it would be in the patient's prone position, you run the risk of the flap being overlaxed when the hip is brought to the flexed position, such as the sitting position. Does it make a difference to you in planning other positioning on the operating table or the ultimate execution of the flap?

DR. STAHL

I think in positioning for a case like this, regardless of the exact position you'd like to place the patient in, you have to make sure that the issue of flexion and positions of maximum stress postoperatively are addressed to make sure you have a secure closure, and what I do is this. No matter what kind of pressure sore I'm doing or what kind of flap I'm using for a given pressure sore, I always will close it in the most taut manner that will be demanded of it postoperatively. For example, with the ischial sores at the time of closure, if I can't close the wound with the hip flexed, then I feel something is wrong and I'm going to try to do more to deliver the tissue more effectively into the wound. I realize that the issue will not have been definitively addressed. So in this particular case, my position would be that I like to do it in a lithotomy position.

Dr. Elliott

The posterior perineum not only includes ischial problems but also the more central posterior perineum, such as the total colectomy wounds with radiation or with neovaginal reconstruction after a total abdominal exenteration or total pelvic exenteration. In that case you've got both coverage and potentially fill, whether it's to fill the wound or to create a neovagina. In addition to the flaps we talked about, the rectus abdominis myocutaneous flap tubed and turned down can sort of serve well for neovaginal reconstruction. I'd also like to point out that using the gracilis, even bilateral gracilis, in this case of filling the depths of a total colectomy-type defect is hazardous because of the distal skin island and arc of rotation.

Dr. Zubowicz

Following up on Dr. Elliott's comment—for those cases that involve the pelvic floor as part of the perineal reconstruction such as the abdominal perineal resection, or a total vaginal hysterectomy, or pelvic exenteration that we are occasionally called to see, I agree strongly that the rectus, with or without a skin paddle, is the ideal solution to the problem. I think that in those circumstances muscles from the leg are severely limited by arcs of rotation. The rectus muscle is an axial flap on its pedicle and can be twisted, turned, and basically be put in a number of positions to take care of the reconstructive list, and anything else would be number 2 way down on the list.

Dr. Toth

The postpelvic exenteration—I think it's important that we remember when we're talking about the rectus, that not uncommonly some of these complex perineal wounds have associated ostomies on the abdomen. Whether it be an ileostomy postexenteration or a urostomy on the opposite side, it's very difficult both in terms of morbidity of donor site and in terms of having the adequate amount of tissue if it were available to get to the perineum. So the rectus not infrequently with some types of perineal reconstruction is not available as an option.

DR. ZUBOWICZ

You don't have to put a stoma through the rectus. We often don't have the choice.

DR. STAHL

Right, that's the problem.

DR. ZUBOWICZ

You're right, but we've done cases where there was an anticipated stoma as part of the extirpation where the reconstruction would be done concurrently, then the plans are made to simply move the stoma out of the way of the rectus that one choses to use. And that solves the problem. I also think that it's important in those cases that you go through adequate preparation of the bowel and so forth to prevent or at least reduce the risk of morbidity from infection.

DR. TOTH

I have one concern about taking the rectus abdominis in a patient who has an ostomy on one side or the other and I see here that it appears as though this is a urostomy, not a cecostomy. But in a patient where abdominal wall integrity is important, I have definite concerns about weakening the abdominal wall, particularly as this patient gets older. In terms of flap selection, I don't see any magic, particularly with regard to muscle, and my choice would have been the inferior gluteal thigh flap, the posterior thigh flap, in terms of being able to bring up an adequate amount of tissue to give you the coverage, to not necessarily have to worry about muscle because we know that the denervated muscle is going to be hard to sort out and provide very little bulk and give you good healthy vascular tissue in the area where you particularly need it.

DR. STAHL

Dr. French, I'm glad you have mentioned the rectus abdominis as a flap for perineal reconstruction. I think it is neglected too often. I share some of the concerns mentioned before, but I think that all in all it is a good flap. I would, for completeness, also mention the possibility of transabdominal transposition of the flap for the central perineal wound, which has been described and can be useful as well, so that it gives this flap even more versatility. Just to bring it through the pelvis for a central perineal wound.

Dr. Elliott

I wanted to follow up on Dr. Toth's comment about using the rectus with a stoma on the abdomen. I've done that a couple of times, even with a colostomy. I have had superficial wound infections when I closed the wound, and if I did that now, again, I would not hesitate to use the rectus for the creation of a neovagina or for a wound such as this, but I would leave the skin open and close it secondarily because I think superficial wound infections are very common in that setting.

Dr. Toth

I am a bit bothered by the fact that in your preoperative planning you elected to take a skin island from a tight abdominal wall and discarded it at the end, and I wonder if in the process of planning whether that need or lack of need could have been anticipated, thereby avoiding the potential complication of wound problems at the skin donor site.

Dr. French

I thought that we would need the skin island, and obviously we didn't, so it was discarded and the muscle was skin grafted. But as far as the closure is concerned, the closure was not unusually tight and I didn't think it compromised the closure by taking out that much of a skin island. And so, I again raised it as a myocutaneous flap, and I have to say I was surprised when I didn't need the skin and subcutaneous portions.

Dr. Grotting

I wanted to ask about a couple of other points and then just make a couple of comments. First of all, maybe you could describe how much fascia you take when you raise it as a vertically oriented myocutaneous flap, how much fascia do you actually need to take. It wasn't quite clear in your description how wide that was. Secondly, then you bring that down and tunnel that subcutaneously. You have to necessarily bring the muscle, or at least the pedicle, through the fascia, and how do you handle the fascial closure around that point where the pedicle comes through when you tunnel it subcutaneously without getting a hernia there? I've had one case where we did in fact get a hernia just exactly at that point. In terms of dropping the muscle transperitoneally, as Dr. Stahl is mentioning, this is another thing that can be problematic in terms of where exactly through the peritoneal cavity you bring it. Obviously, you can get good closure of the anterior fascia when you drop everything inside, but dealing with the femoral canal or if you're bringing it through the obturator canal, for example, these are other areas that are prone to herniation. Also the use of this flap in a young woman, and as I'm sure you're aware, this muscle flap can be harvested through an abdominoplasty approach and if you did require a skin graft, your point about using the overlying skin island, that can be handled by removing a little skin with the abdominoplasty-type closure and using that as a donor site that can be closed primarily.

Dr. French

Regarding your question about the amount of fascia that's taken: it's just the fascia that essentially is beneath the skin island. If the skin island extends medially over the midline, obviously that's not a problem. It's basically the perforators that come up right beneath that skin island. I hope that answers your question. But that's all we did on this particular flap. As for where we take it through the fascia, it's more inferolaterally. This patient did not get a hernia and I don't know of any hernias that we've had from that, but I certainly can understand what you're saying. It is certainly a possibility.

REFERENCES

1. Taylor GI, Corlett R, Boyd JB. Extended deep inferior epigastric flap: A clinical technique. Plast Reconstr Surg 1983;72:751.

2. Pena MM, Stephenson G, Smith SJ, Given KS. The inferiorly-based rectus abdominis myocutaneous flap for reconstruction of recurrent pressure sore. Plast Reconstr Surg 1992;89:90.

Hartrampf CR, Sheflan M, Black PW. Breast reconstruction with a transverse abdominal island flap. Plast Reconstr Surg 1982;69:216.

Mathes SJ, Nahai F. Clinical Atlas of Muscle and Musculocutaneous flaps. St. Louis: Mosby, 1979.

Tobin GR, Day TG. Vaginal and pelvic reconstruction with distally-based myocutaneous flap. Plast Reconstr Surg 1988;81:62.

Gottlieb ME, Chandrasekhar B, Terz JJ, Sherman R. Clinical applications of the extended deep inferior epigastric flap. Plast Reconstr Surg 1986;78:782.

Boyd JB, Taylor GI, Corlett R. Vascular territories of the superior epigastric and deep inferior epigastric systems. Plast Reconstr Surg 1984;73:1.

Bunkis J, Fudem GM. Rectus abdominis flap closure of ischial sacral pressure sore. Ann Plast Surg 1989;23:447.

Bostwick J. Plastic and Reconstructive Breast Surgery. Quality Medical Publishing Inc., 1990.

7

Decision Making
in
Lower Extremity
Reconstruction

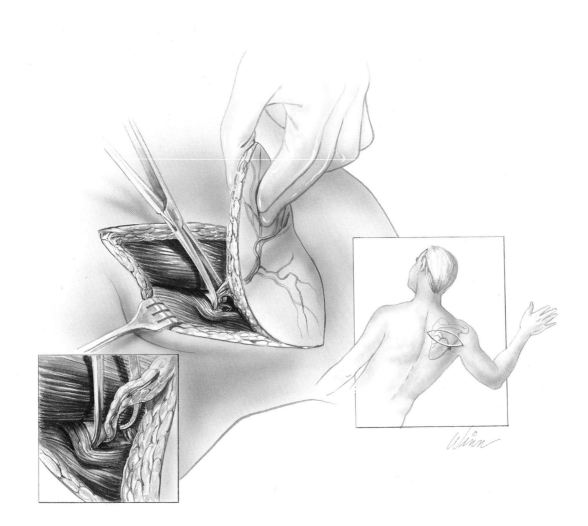

SCAPULAR FREE FLAP

L. FRANKLYN ELLIOTT

THE PROBLEM

This 15-year-old girl was referred to us with a history of previously diagnosed ulcerative colitis and weight loss. She had been on sulfasalazine and prednisone, and at the time we were consulted she was admitted with multifocal osteomyelitis of the left leg associated with open wounds. The ulcerative colitis had been diagnosed 2 years prior to admission and had been quiescent for approximately 1 year. There were two foci of osteomyelitis diagnosed on bone scan with positive cultures for *Staphylococcus*. These were located in the proximal medial tibia and the lateral malleolus. Debridement of these two wounds was performed by the orthopedic service, and the patient was presented to us with open wounds involving exposed bone and history of osteomyelitis (Figure 13.1).

INTRODUCTION

A recent perusal of two significant reviews of lower extremity reconstruction reveals no fewer than 29 suggested reconstructive options in the

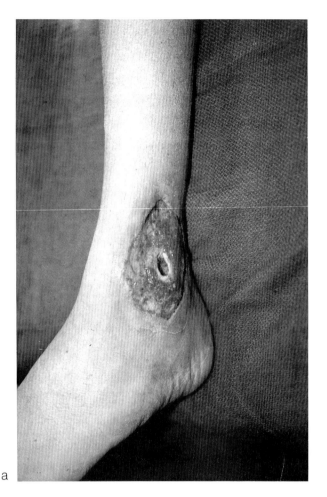
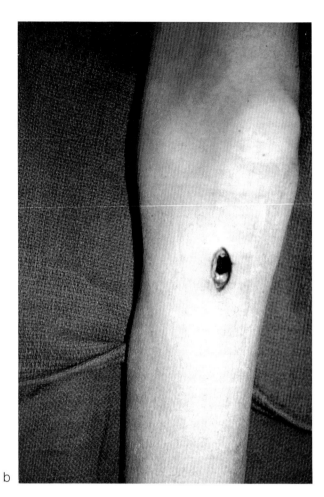

a   b

Figure 13.1. (a) Preoperative view of left lateral ankle with exposure of malleolus and loss of cortical bone. (b) Second focus of osteomyelitis in proximal left tibia. This was closed with a local flap.

lower leg and foot in one source and 20 options in another.[1,2] This is an enormous smorgasbord from which to choose. There is no question that many of the different flaps are specifically indicated for certain problems. There are a number of wound characteristics that dictate a specific flap choice. Some of these are the location of the wound (upper, middle, or lower third of the tibia, ankle, or foot), size of the wound, exposure of bone with or without associated dead space, need for bone replacement, presence or absence of weight-bearing surface, age, life-style, and even gender of the patient. With this myriad of wound characteristics in mind, it is obvious that one cannot be too dogmatic in suggesting a single flap for all lower leg and foot problems requiring flap reconstruction. Nonetheless, this chapter will focus on two flap choices that appear to have versatility in responding to a wide range of wounds, success rates that compare with any flap choice, and aesthetic results that are compatible with the demands of microsurgery in the 1990s.

It is always wise to consider the reconstructive ladder[3] in devising the appropriate reconstructive response to any open wound, particularly in the lower leg and foot. But coverage alone is not always enough, particularly in the lower extremity, when bone is involved. The second element for success in the *cure* of a complex wound of the lower extremity is adequate debridement, which demands the removal of bacterial contamination or infection from the wound or underlying bone. These two elements—debridement and well-vascularized coverage—go hand in hand in creating the dramatic increase in percentages of cure in these complex problems noted from World War I to World War II to today.[4,5] There have been numerous significant advances in the care of these patients over the past century, including antisepsis, debridement, overall patient stabilization and resuscitation, antibiotics, stabilization of the extremity, and rehabilitation. These will not be recounted here. We will chiefly focus on the reconstruction aspect, highlighting the most refined method of reconstructing certain complex soft tissue wounds of the lower extremity, ankle, and foot today by the scapular free fascial flap.

The patient in Figure 13.1 needs well-vascularized flap tissue for coverage of the open ankle wound. There was a history of osteomyelitis with exposed bone in a cachectic patient who had been suffering from chronic ulcerative colitis. The tissues around the ankle and foot for rotation are sparse in most patients but were deemed particularly unsuitable in this patient, with her underlying medical problems. For these two reasons, a free flap coverage was felt to be necessary. The requirements for the flap are that there is excellent blood flow in the transferred tissue and that there is thin but durable coverage. Furthermore, the donor site scar should be minimal in this young patient.

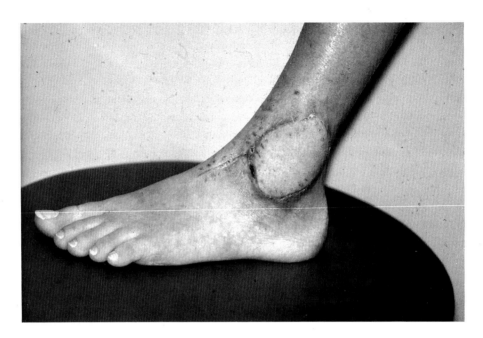

Figure 13.2. One-year postoperative scapula free flap to ankle.

The free scapular flap was performed on this patient without complications. She was discharged on the eighth postoperative day. After 1 year (Figure 13.2) she has no evidence of recurrence of her osteomyelitis, and the wound remains healed.

ANATOMY

The scapular and parascapular flaps were first described and detailed in the early 1980s by Dos Santos and Nassif.[7,8] Both of these flaps were described as cutaneous free flaps based on the extensive circulation of the blood vessels lying over the dorsal surface of the scapula and emanating at or near the trilateral space as the circumflex scapular vessels (Figure 13.3). The trilateral space is bounded by the teres minor superiorly, the teres major inferiorly, and the long head of the triceps laterally. There are generally two main branches of the circumflex scapular vessels as they leave the trilateral space and supply the upper to middle back. These vessels are

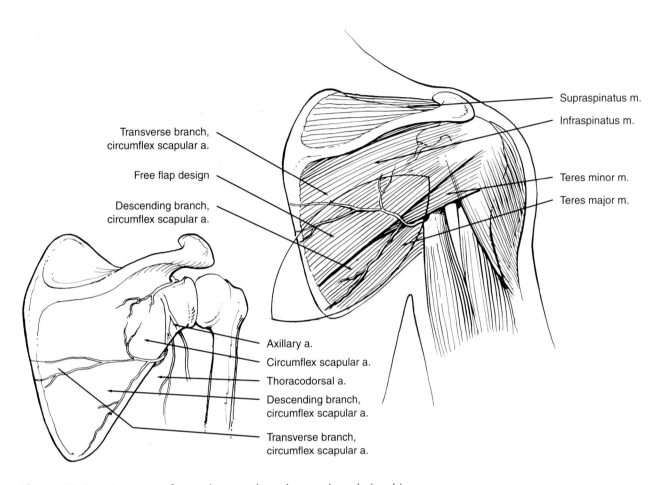

Transverse branch, circumflex scapular a.

Free flap design

Descending branch, circumflex scapular a.

Supraspinatus m.

Infraspinatus m.

Teres minor m.

Teres major m.

Axillary a.

Circumflex scapular a.

Thoracodorsal a.

Descending branch, circumflex scapular a.

Transverse branch, circumflex scapular a.

Figure 13.3.   Anatomy of scapular vessels and muscular relationship.

located along the lateral border of the scapula and over the mid-transverse portion of the scapula, respectively. They are generally known as the parascapular and scapular branches. From these two branches come the names "parascapular" and "scapular" flaps. Both of these flaps have proven to be robust in blood supply, minimal in donor site deficit, and versatile in size and shape.[9-11]

It is apparent that these two flaps are not necessarily distinct but are part of a wide territory of back skin that can be supplied either by fascio-cutaneous perforators from the circumflex scapular system or by musculo-cutaneous perforators from the latissimus dorsi muscle (thoracodorsal pedicle) (Figure 13.3). These systems are so extensive that the scapular flap has been found to reliably extend superiorly to the spine of the scapula, medially across the midline, inferiorly to the posterior iliac crest (when the latissimus dorsi is included), and laterally to at least the mid-axillary line.

The blood vessels of this flap are essentially microscopic over much of the broad expanse of the flap. As the vessels make their way toward the lateral border of the scapula, they begin to coalesce into larger channels, so that they can be visualized within the fascia. The vessels finally converge as the transverse scapular branch and the parascapular branch to form the circumflex scapular artery. The circumflex scapular artery varies in diameter from 2 to 3 mm, with generally a single accompanying vein. Once formed, the circumflex scapular vessels wrap around the lateral border of the scapula and penetrate deep to the scapula to join the thoracodorsal artery and form the subscapular artery. The length of the circumflex scapular artery is 3 to 5 cm. The length of the entire pedicle is reported as being 5.5 to 10 cm.[12] This length can be attained only by including portions of the transverse scapular or parascapular branches as part of the pedicle.

An added refinement to the scapular free flap is the harvest of the fascia alone with its blood supply and without overlying skin.[13] In dissecting the scapular fascia flap, the skin, its subdermal plexus, and a layer of underlying fat (to preserve the subdermal plexus) are elevated over the remaining underlying superficial and deep fascia, thus leaving this underlying layer undisturbed while maintaining blood supply to the overlying elevated skin.[5] The deep fascia can then be elevated from the underlying epimysium of the muscles which surround, support, and envelop the scapula bone, creating a thin flap which is extremely well vascularized because of the size of the vessels flowing into the flap and the significant arborization throughout the fascia (Figure 13.4). This fascial flap does, however, lack overlying skin coverage.

The indications for the scapular free flap are reflected by the anatomy as described above. It is indicated for any wound with exposed bone or tendon of the lower extremity, ankle, and foot in which excessive bulk and contour is a potential problem, whether it is functional or aesthetic. It is,

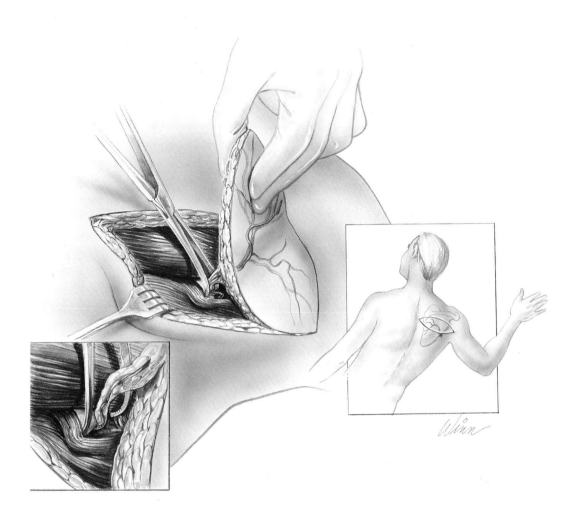

Figure 13.4. Elevation of scapular flap. Inset A: Design of skin paddle. Inset B: Detail of pedicle as it comes around lateral scapular border.

therefore, indicated specifically for those wounds of the anterior, medial, and lateral tibia, the medial or lateral malleolus, and the foot/heel—either the plantar or the posterior surfaces. These wounds account for a significant percentage of lower extremity wounds for which plastic surgeons are consulted. They are characterized by the need for thin, pliable, well-vascularized soft tissue coverage that will restore the contour of the injured extremity while providing well-vascularized soft tissue to address the underlying demands of the potentially ischemic and/or contaminated bone.

TECHNIQUE

Preoperatively, the most important landmarks to delineate are the outline of the body of the scapula, including the scapula tip and the spine of the scapula. This is usually done with the patient in a sitting position. The relationship between the spine of the scapula and the tip of the scapula gives a precise location of the trilateral space and therefore the scapular vessels. The location of the circumflex scapular vessels at the lateral border of the scapula is that point which is two-thirds up the lateral border of the scapula from the tip of the scapula to the spine of the scapula. The skin flap can then be designed depending on the needs at the recipient site overlying either the parascapular vessels or the scapular vessels or both.

If the defect is on the medial aspect of the lower extremity or foot, then the opposite-side scapular flap is utilized. Conversely, if there is a lateral defect and one is using the peroneal vessel as a recipient vessel, then the ipsilateral scapular flap is used.

The proposed flap size can be decided upon using a template created from the recipient site defect and transposed to the operative site on the back. It is not necessary to make the flap any larger than the defect, even though the flap will appear smaller because of secondary retraction once it is elevated. However, once transferred, the flap can again be stretched out to its initial dimensions and cover the defect completely.

The most medial portions of the incisions are first made and the flap is elevated just superficial to the investing fascia of the underlying musculature. The flap is elevated rather rapidly in this deep layer up over the lower one-third of the scapula. Vessels on the deep surface of the flap will begin to become apparent as elevation proceeds toward the lateral border of the scapula. These vessels form the first macroscopic portions of the scapular vascular system and converge to form the circumflex scapular vessels at the midportion of the lateral border of the scapula.

The entire incision is now completed, continuing laterally toward the axilla. The flap remains attached by an accumulation of fat along the lateral border of the scapula encircling the circumflex scapular vessels. The muscles bordering the triangular space are identified, thus defining the triangular space. However, the vessels generally remain encased in a fat packet, which makes their identification not readily apparent except in the thinnest patient. Dissection of the vessels at this point is best done using loupe magnification. Several techniques can help in identifying the location of the main vessels. The first of these is to locate a vessel of 1 to 2 mm in diameter and trace it to the main channel of the circumflex scapular vessels. Another is to completely bypass the fat packet at the lateral border of the scapula and simply retract the teres major superiorly and the latissimus dorsi inferiorly. This will allow access deeper into the triangular space and identification of the vessels proximal to it. It is a bit more difficult to try to identify this pedicle by continuing to elevate the flap laterally and explore along the lateral border of the scapula, since there are numerous small branches that dive behind the lateral border of the scapula that are difficult to manage if the pedicle has not been identified (Figure 13.4, Inset B). Once the circumflex scapular pedicle is identified, the flap is a complete island flap. It is preferable to include both the transverse and the descending scapular branches, since this will increase the vascularity of the overall flap, but it is clear that the flap will survive on either of these branches.

The circumflex scapular vessels can now be dissected for varying lengths, depending on the pedicle length demands at the recipient site. This dissection is probably the most tedious part of the flap dissection. The circumflex scapular vessels traced to the takeoff of the thoracodorsal vessels give a length of 5 to 6 cm. If extra length is required, dissection continues proximal to the takeoff of the thoracodorsal vessels, but the dissection becomes quite deep and difficult. Nonetheless, with proper retraction the vessels can be dissected to the axillary vessels, creating a long pedicle of 7 to 10 cm.

At the recipient site, the condition of the vessels varies significantly when one compares the acute setting with that of the delayed or chronic complex open wound of the lower extremity. The delayed or chronic wound is characterized by significant scarring in all planes, reflecting extensive damage often associated with the force needed to create massive wounds of the lower extremity. The biologic resolution of this force is scarring within muscles, along tendons, and along neurovascular bundles. With regard to a microsurgical tissue transfer, this scarring is most significant in association with the blood vessels. It results in disappearance of normal dissection planes between the structures of the neurovascular bundle, thickening of the adventitia of the blood vessels leading to difficulty in differentiation between the adventitia and the media, a profound tendency toward vasospasm, particularly in the artery, and friability of the intima. For these reasons, it is always preferable to extend the incisions out of the zone of injury if possible. Here these changes will begin to disappear and the situation returns to a more normal state. However, the farther the dissection is from the wound, the longer the pedicle that is needed. Vein grafts to extend the pedicle out of the zone of injury are not a great problem on the arterial side but can be of more concern in the low-flow veins.

It is almost always preferable to perform an arterial anastomosis in the lower extremity in an end-to-side manner unless the extreme distal extent of one of the three arteries of the lower leg or foot is used. Prograde perfusion is preserved at the same time as the flap is vascularized. The venous anastomosis is generally performed in an end-to-end manner, assuming that size discrepancy does not exceed 2 to 1. There is some argument for end-to-side anastomoses on the venous side, since this technique may ensure greater blood flow through the veins when both prograde and flap flow are combined. However, flap flow is usually so robust that the end-to-end anastomosis on the venous side appears to be as successful as the end-to-side technique.

The flap can be sewn in to cover the defect either before or after the vascular anastomoses are performed. We generally inset the flap after the flap is revascularized so that any kinking of the vessels can be observed as the flap is placed down over the wound. One should not be reluctant to stretch out the flap to its normal dimensions, because this tightness will not threaten the survival of the flap but will prevent redundancy of the flap and provide a better contour once healing has occurred.

Postoperatively, we do not routinely transfer patients to the intensive care unit after a free flap transfer. On the other hand, frequent monitoring of the donor and recipient sites by nurses and/or physicians is characteristic of the postoperative care in these patients. Although many options exist for the sophisticated monitoring of the flap, we have opted for direct inspection by the doctor or a trained nurse as the best technique to date. Our technique for monitoring involved frequent inspections of the flap by the physician over the first 12 to 18 hours postoperatively. The key to this or any other monitoring technique is that if there is any suspicion of a problem, then immediate return to the operating room is mandatory. It cannot be overemphasized how successful salvage of a flap can be if it occurs early, and how unsuccessful it is if stasis or coagulation is allowed to remain in recently transferred tissue. If there is access to the vascular pedicle, it can receive direct Doppler examination, another objective assessment of continued blood flow to the flap. However, it must be clear that one is examining the *flap* vessel and not the native leg vessel.

DISCUSSION

The scapular free flap is an excellent choice for coverage of complex lower extremity injuries that are referred to plastic surgeons. The flap is thin, but potentially quite large, and can be harvested in a myriad of shapes to satisfy the needs at the recipient site. The vessels are long, constant, and relatively easily dissected. There is no disruption of the musculoskeletal function that characterizes the harvest of other muscle flaps. For these reasons, the scapular free flap compares favorably to some of the other leading choices, including the latissimus or segmental latissimus muscle flap, the gracilis free flap, or the temporoparietal fascial flap. The temporoparietal fascial flap is limited in size and does not have overlying skin coverage. It is also a more bloody dissection with a pedicle that can be as long, but, if so, requires a more difficult dissection along the mandibular ramus.

As with any other flap, there are potential pitfalls and complications with the use of the scapular flap. If the skin island needed is too large to allow easy closure on the back, significant spreading of the scar on the back, or even dehiscence of the wound can occur. In some cases, it is necessary to skin graft the back when large scapular free flaps are used. This creates a relatively unsightly donor defect, which can be improved with tissue expansion secondarily but probably in most cases, would cause the surgeon to think of other donor sites if a flap this size is warranted. On the other hand, appropriate sources of large amounts of thin flap skin are fairly limited, since generally the abdominal wall skin is associated with a panniculus which is much thicker than that of the scapular flap.

The obese patient presents several specific considerations when a free scapular flap is harvested. The identification of the scapular vessels at the lateral scapular border may also be more difficult, since there is a considerable amount of adipose tissue in the triangular space. Dissection in these patients must be more deliberate so as to clearly identify the scapular vessels themselves and not just a feeding vessel. The prepping and draping of the upper extremity and of the wound on the side of the flap harvest is a helpful adjunct to allow better exposure in the posterior axillary region. Since the scapular vessels are characterized by numerous tiny feeding vessels as they travel around the lateral border of the scapula, it is probably better to plan the flap more distally on the back to allow a longer pedicle and not require the dissection of the pedicle around the lateral border and deep to the scapula. Finally, the obese patient may have inappropriate thickness of the scapular flap when the overlying skin is included. In this setting a scapular *fascial* free flap might be a better choice, transferring the flap without overlying skin and subsequently skin grafting the fascial free flap on the recipient site.

ROUNDTABLE DISCUSSION

DR. ELLIOTT

The scapular free flap was chosen for the reasons enumerated in this chapter. Refinements in lower extremity reconstruction are clearly possible as we have improved our microvascular techniques over the past 20 years. Thin, well-vascularized coverage is most similar to what is missing in these open wounds of the lower third of the tibia, ankle, and foot. Therefore, a flap such as the scapular free flap will be the standard against which other flaps are evaluated.

DR. GROTTING

I have several questions which I think would be worth discussing. First, you mentioned using the scapular fascial flap without overlying skin. Do you think that is as durable and equally as good aesthetically? Second, should we consider the possibility of adding sensation in an area where there will be continued friction and breakdown, not because of the durability of coverage, but because of insensate tissue?

DR. ELLIOTT

The transfer of a scapular flap without overlying skin was mentioned with regard to the obese patient, in whom a transfer of the full-thickness flap would yield a thicker, possibly more unacceptable flap.[12,13] I do agree, though, that skin-grafted fascia, especially within the first year, is going to be less durable than a full-thickness flap which includes overlying skin.

With regard to sensation, I don't think that fine cutaneous sensation is generally achievable at this point. The sensation on which most patients depend, I believe, is deep sensibility transferred through the flap to the bone or deep tissues. One must have a cooperative and understanding patient, particularly in the first year or so after reconstruction, to prevent overuse of the area and subsequent breakdown. After this period of time, it is generally a combination of the patient being aware of the area, along with the return of deep sensibility, which helps to prevent subsequent breakdown.

DR. STAHL

One flap that was not mentioned is the radial forearm flap. There is probably an increased potential for sensibility with this flap, though the disadvantages include the appearance and possible morbidity of the donor site. Repair of the forearm free flap donor site has improved, though, over the past few years (Figure 13.5) and therefore can be minimized. I also think that the foot should be differentiated from the leg. Personally, I like the rectus abdominis with skin grafts for the more longitudinal, proximal leg reconstruction.

DR. ZUBOWICZ

I would have chosen a different approach to this problem, using a gracilis muscle with a skin graft. I think it is important that we consider in the 1990s the price to the patient in terms of donor site morbidity. This is particularly a consideration in the younger patient, who is more likely to expose the back. The donor morbidity from the gracilis flap is extraordinarily low unless one happens to be a bullfrog. The scar is very inconspicuous and the operation is quite easy. A second aspect of this flap is the concept that a muscle does a better job in mopping up bacteria than a skin fascial flap. I would like to know your thoughts on this theory.

DR. MOSES

If you are going to use a fascial flap for a smaller wound, why not use a temporoparietal flap, since the donor site scar is completely hidden? I realize that the scapular flap can provide a much larger potential surface, but in this case why not use a scar that would be completely hidden?

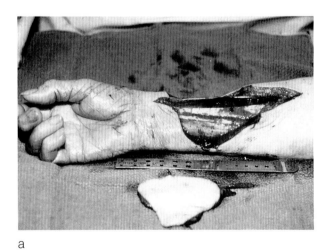
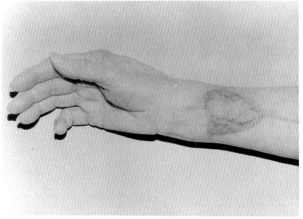

a   b

Figure 13.5. Donor defect site of radial forearm flap. (a) Defect at time of dissection. (b) Defect 1 year later after skin graft.

DR. TOTH

The concept of cushioning has been brought up, particularly on weight-bearing surfaces. I am concerned about the concept of a purely fascial flap without overlying skin, in view of the traditional difficulty of getting skin grafts to heal directly over fat. I would have chosen a different flap—the free serratus flap. It would also provide thin pliable tissue, cushioning, and reliability of a skin graft healing over a vascular muscle as opposed to overvascularized fat.

DR. MCKINNON

I agree with Dr. Moses that the temporal parietal free flap would have been a better choice due to vessel size and consistent success.

DR. ELLIOTT

I still use the temporalis free flap, but in my experience it is limited in size. In addition, I find the dissection of it definitely more difficult than that of the scapular flap. There is more blood loss and the risk of alopecia. I have not had a problem with alopecia and the temporalis free flap, but the potential is there. Another problem with the temporalis free flap is pedicle length. Clearly, it can be dissected for an extensive length. However, the further one dissects it inferiorly, the further it drops behind the mandible, making the dissection more difficult.

The cushioning effect was mentioned with regard to a muscle, but I don't believe the specialized tissue of muscle is a better cushion than that of fat. In fact, most bony prominences are covered with a sliding surface of fat and skin, not muscle. Furthermore, muscle does atrophy and the cushion thins. The fat, however, should remain at its transferred thickness.

Grafting on fat has not been as successful as grafting on muscle, and one must keep this in mind if a purely fascial scapular free flap is chosen. I would probably not choose this flap for a weight-bearing surface.

DR. MOSES

We have not mentioned the use of arteriography prior to free flap reconstruction of the lower extremity. In the case of this adolescent patient, arteriography would be less of a consideration, but in the older, more complicated patient, I think an arteriogram would be a good idea preoperatively.

DR. GROTTING

I agree that arteriography should be considered in most patients prior to free flap reconstruction of the lower extremity, for two reasons. The first is the status of the vessels proximal to the wound, and the second is the overall blood supply to the foot, in case your plan for a recipient vessel choice does not work. If an end-to-side anastomosis must be converted to an end-to-end anastomosis, you should know the overall blood supply to the foot to be comfortable with transecting one of three main arteries. In addition, if one has to shift from the dorsalis pedis artery to the posterior tibial artery, it is again helpful to know arterial dominance and the location of any proximal arterial lesions.

DR. ELLIOTT

My approach towards an arteriogram prior to free flap coverage of the lower extremity is that I don't routinely do it. If it is a younger patient and the pulses are present, I generally don't obtain an arteriogram. I think arteriograms are not as accurate and as informative as we might think. Direct observation under the microscope is better. I have had a number of occasions in the past where an arteriogram suggested tiny and unusable vessels, but on dissection the vessels were found to be adequate. On the other hand, with foot reconstruction problems, it is wise to have a working knowledge of the collateral flow in the foot so that several options might be available.

Finally, there is clearly a role for arteriography in the older patient who might have proximal disease or in the patient in whom one suspects previously damaged vessels due to trauma.

DR. GROTTING

With regard to sensation, I feel we are reaching the point where we can restore sensibility where sensibility has been lost by direct nerve coaptation. Under these circumstances, I would try to pick a flap where we have a potential to restore cutaneous sensibility. In this circumstance, the superficial branch of the peroneal nerve or perhaps the sural nerve might have been an option.

I have largely abandoned the temporoparietal fascial flap because of the unpredictability of the donor vessels, particularly the vein, and because this flap tends to atrophy to the point of becoming almost nonexistent.

References

1. Strauch B, Vasconez LO, Hall-Findley EJ. Encyclopedia of Flaps III. Boston: Little, Brown & Co., 1990.

2. Byrd HS. Lower extremity reconstruction. Select Read Plast Surg 1992;6:1–27.

3. Mathes SJ, Nahai F. Clinical applications for Muscle and Musculocutaneous Flaps. St. Louis: C.V. Mosby Co., 1982.

4. Burklatter WE. Open injuries of the lower extremity. Surg Clin North Am 1973;53:1439.

5. Aldea PA, Shaw WW. The evolution of the surgical management of severe lower extremity trauma. Clin Plast Surg 1986;13:549.

6. dos Santos LF. Dos retalho eslapular: Un novo retalho livre microcirurgico. Rev Bras Circ 1980;70:133.

7. Nassif TM, Vidal L, Boret JL, Baudet J. The parascapular flap: A new cutaneous microsurgical free flap. Plast Reconstr Surg 1982;69:59.

8. Gilbert A, Teot L. The free scapular flap. Plast Reconstr Surg 1982;69:601.

9. Vrbamath JR, Koman LA, Goldmer RD, Armstrong NB, Nunley JA. The vascularized cutaneous scapular flap. Plast Reconstr Surg 1982;69:772.

10. Barwick WJ, Goodkind DJ, Serafin D. The free scapular flap. Plast Reconstr Surg 1982;69:779.

11. Kim PS, Gottlieb JR, Harris GD, Nagle DJ, Lewis VL. The dorsal thoracic fascia: Anatomic significance with clinical applications in reconstructive microsurgery. Plast Reconstr Surg 1987;79:72.

12. Chen D, Jupiter JB, Lipton HA, Li S. The parascapular flap for treatment of lower extremity disorders. Plast Reconstr Surg 1989;84:108.

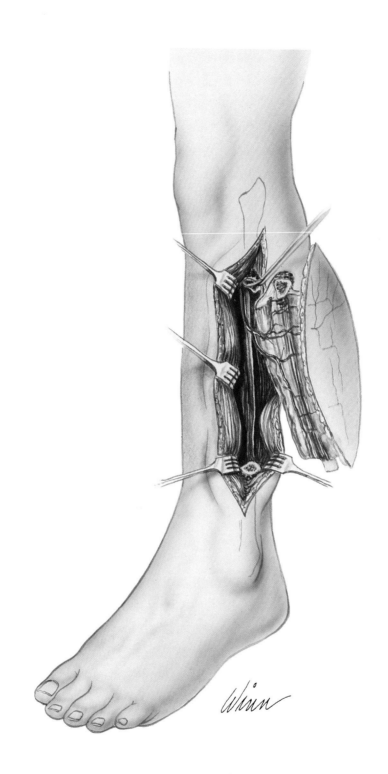

FREE FIBULA RECONSTRUCTION

L. FRANKLYN ELLIOTT

THE PROBLEM

This 34-year-old man sustained a severe crush injury to the left lower extremity when a forklift fell on that extremity. He presented to us approximately 1 week after the injury and after initial debridement. There was a large, full-thickness skin-loss open wound of the anteromedial aspect of the distal third of the tibia with exposed tibia (Figure 14.1).

This was initially treated successfully using a microvascular free latissimus dorsi muscle transfer and split-thickness skin graft (Figure 14.2). Approximately 10 months later, he presented with redness in the upper portions of the tibial wound with the presence of persistent internal fixation devices and a nonunion. At the time of debridement, there was a nonunion approximately 18 to 20 cm above the ankle mortis along with two inferiorly placed butterfly fragments which were not healed. All of this area was segmentally debrided without evidence of viable bone. This created a gap in the tibia of some 12 cm.

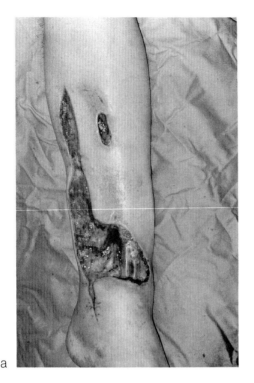

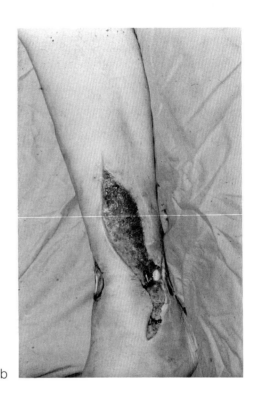

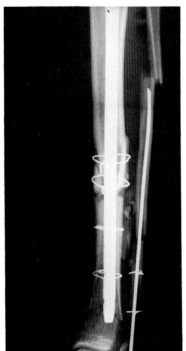

Figure 14.1. (a) Presenting open wound of left distal tibia, medial view. (b) Lateral view. (c) Radiograph of initial injury.

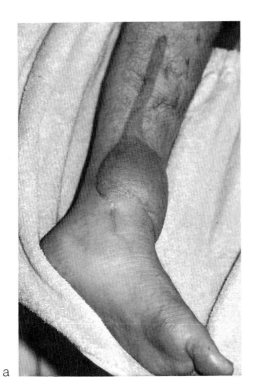
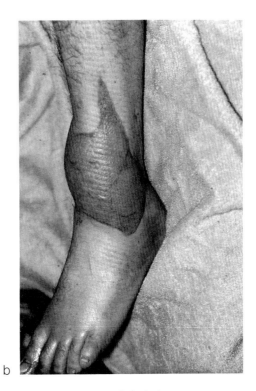

a b

Figure 14.2. Healed wound of lower extremity after coverage with latissimus free flap and skin graft. (a) Medial view. (b) Lateral view.

Introduction

Lower-extremity reconstruction becomes more complex when there are absent segments of bone as opposed to only exposed healthy or healing bone.[6] As with soft tissue defects, debridement of any necrotic or infected tissue is a mainstay in achieving cure. With the absence of a segment of bone, stabilization becomes paramount in achieving a successful outcome. After complete debridement and solid fixation with healthy overlying soft tissue coverage and underlying periosteum, primary healing will occur without corticocancellous bone grafts. This is true for defects less than 6 cm. For defects greater than 6 cm, restoration of the bony defect is best performed using vascularized bone graft.[16] Defects from 6 to 30 cm can be bridged using a free bone flap from one of several sites.

The addition of the Ilizarov bone transit technique[14,15] has added to our options for managing difficult bony problems of the lower extremity. The Ilizarov technique of bone transportation has proven to be faster in healing, safer in the compromised host, and cheaper in terms of operative time and hospitalization for those defects less than 6 cm which otherwise could be treated with bone grafting. The Ilizarov technique is being expanded into defects larger than 6 cm, but at this date vascularized bone flaps are still first choice for defects greater than 6 cm.

The indications for free fibula flap are bony defects greater than 6 cm after trauma, tumor resection, or congenital abnormality of the tibia (pseudoarthrosis). The advantages of the free fibula are that: it is of varying length and can be sectioned to meet the defect needs; it is of appropriate caliber so as to fit snugly within the medullary cavity of the recipient tibia; it can be harvested under tourniquet control, producing minimal blood loss; it has a long and constant vascular pedicle and can be harvested with or without associated muscle or overlying skin island. Though other choices remain for vascularized bone graft—iliac crest, scapula bone flap—the free fibula remains the transfer of choice in the majority of cases of bony defects in the tibia greater than 6 cm.[17]

Due to the length of this defect, a free fibula flap with overlying skin island was harvested from the right leg and transferred to the left leg. The fibula bone was intercalated into the tibial gap and additional bone graft was placed (Figure 14.3). The free fibula was revascularized by sewing into the thoracodorsal vessels of the previous latissimus free flap. The flap healed without complication or subsequent infection. However, the distal bone junction did require additional bone grafting 1 year later to fill in a fibrous union. Now, 3 years postoperatively, he has complete bone union and reconstitution of the extremity (Figure 14.4).

Anatomy

The free fibula flap is supplied by the peroneal vessels, which are part of the trifurcation of the popliteal artery just distal to the knee. Generally the

Figure 14.3. Radiograph after debridement and insertion of fibula.

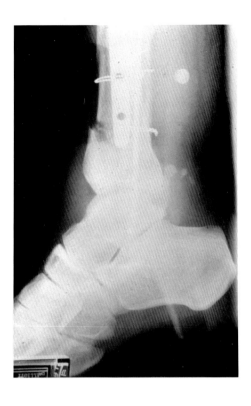

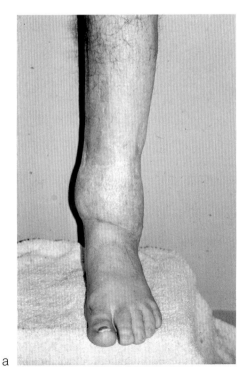

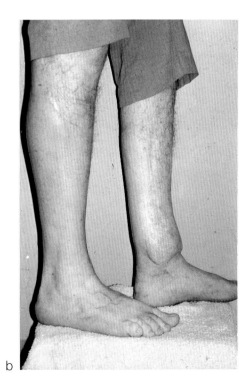

a   b

Figure 14.4. Three years after initial injury. (a) Frontal view. (b) Medial view.

anterior tibial artery takes off initially and passes cephalad to the interosseous membrane at the proximal fibula head (Figure 14.5). The other portion of the vessel divides at a varying distance of 1 to 3 cm to become the posterior tibial artery medially and the peroneal artery laterally. The peroneal artery runs posterior to the interosseous membrane in the substance of the flexor hallucis longus muscle. It supplies perforating branches into the adjacent musculature, including the flexor hallucis longus, the peroneus longus and brevis, and portions of the soleus muscle. It also provides periosteal branches that supply the fibula, the septocutaneous vessels which run between the peroneal group and the soleus muscle, and the musculocutaneous vessels through the soleus to the skin. The main channel of the peroneal artery continues to within 3 to 4 cm of the lateral ankle, where it generally becomes quite small and terminates in some patients as the lateral calcaneal artery.

The blood supply of the fibula is chiefly via the periosteum. The peroneal artery provides blood flow for the periosteum of the distal two-thirds

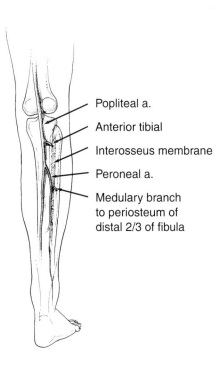

Popliteal a.

Anterior tibial

Interosseus membrane

Peroneal a.

Medulary branch to periosteum of distal 2/3 of fibula

Figure 14.5. Vascular anatomy of free fibula flap.

of the bone and the anterior tibial artery for the proximal one-third of the bone. The peroneal artery has a distinct medullary artery into the fibula that is generally located at the junction of the proximal one-third and distal two-thirds of the fibula.

The fibula is a straight bone with a thick, dense cortex and a small medullary cavity. The bone widens at the proximal and distal ends and becomes an important component of stabilization of both the knee and the ankle. The lower end of the fibula forms the lateral malleolus, and the proximal end supports knee stability through fibular collateral ligaments to the tibia. The central portion of the fibula is attached to the tibia via the interosseous membrane (Figure 14.6).

There are three muscle compartments of the thigh—the anterior, lateral, and posterior. The anterior compartment is confined by the tibia medially and the lateral compartment laterally. It contains the tibialis anterior, extensor digitorum longus, extensor hallucis longus, and peroneus tertius. The anterior compartment also contains the anterior tibial neurovascular bundle, which lies deep to the tibialis anterior on the interosseous membrane approximately 1 cm medial to the fibula. These muscles are innervated by the deep peroneal nerve. The lateral compartment is made up of the peroneus longus and brevis and is tightly confined between two interosseous membranes. The posterior compartment has a superficial and deep portion. The deep portion contains the flexor hallucis and tibialis posterior muscles, the former rising from the posterior surface of the fibula. The superficial portion contains the soleus, gastrocnemius, and plantaris muscles. Of the three members of the superficial portion of the posterior compartment, only the soleus muscle has a direct attachment to the fibula.

The tibial nerve divides into the common peroneal nerve and the posterior tibial nerve in the popliteal fossa. The peroneal nerve is particularly important with regard to the free fibula dissection, since it courses around the lateral head of the fibula to divide into the deep and superficial peroneal nerves. The deep peroneal nerve accompanies the anterior tibial vessels on the anterior surface of the interosseous membrane and supplies the muscles of the anterior compartment. The superficial peroneal nerve re-

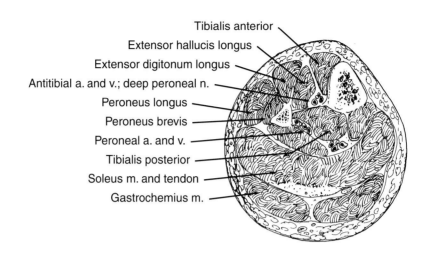

Tibialis anterior
Extensor hallucis longus
Extensor digitonum longus
Antitibial a. and v.; deep peroneal n.
Peroneus longus
Peroneus brevis
Peroneal a. and v.
Tibialis posterior
Soleus m. and tendon
Gastrochemius m.

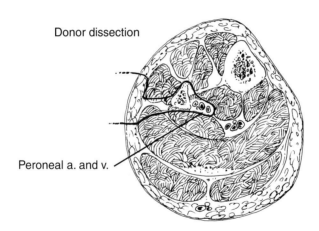

Donor dissection

Peroneal a. and v.

Figure 14.6. Muscular relationships to fibula.

mains subcutaneous and supplies sensation to the dorsum of the foot. Injury to the common peroneal nerve can occur during the proximal incision for harvesting of the free fibula flap, and this should be avoided. Injury to the deep peroneal nerve should also be avoided so that dorsiflexion of the foot will be maintained. The amount of muscle taken with the free fibula will determine whether or not the superficial peroneal nerve can be maintained, since the superficial peroneal nerve runs just superficial to the peroneal group.

Technique

The patient is best positioned in a lateral decubitus position with the leg from which the fibula is to be harvested turned up. Skin preparation is continued above the popliteal fossa just posterior to the lateral head of the fibula and then along the lateral aspect of the leg for whatever distance is necessary to harvest the necessary skin island and underlying bone. The initial incision defines the *posterior* perimeter of the skin island. The location of the bone harvest depends on the length of bone needed and the length of the pedicle needed. For instance, if a shorter bony length is needed, it can be taken more distally on the fibula, thus giving a longer peroneal artery length after its takeoff from the posterior tibial artery until it joins the graft portion of the fibula. On the other hand, if the fibula length is greater, the pedicle length may be necessarily less because the fibula will be harvested more proximally. The overlying skin island should be centered over the membranous septum which separates the lateral and posterior compartments. This is the location of the largest and most predictable perforators providing cutaneous blood flow from the peroneal artery. These vessels can be located with the use of Doppler ultrasonography. On the other hand, the island can be centered over the palpable lateral edge of the fibula, which will ensure incorporation of the underlying perforators. A skin island 5 to 7 cm in width is all that is generally possible if primary closure is desired. The incision continues deeper, reflecting the lateral gastrocnemius posteriorly. The lateral soleus origin on the fibula is dissected posteriorly under tourniquet control using the Bovie, leaving a small cuff of soleus muscle on the lateral fibula. This exposes the popliteal fossa and the neurovascular bundles in the proximal leg.

The most common vascular anatomy is an anterior tibial artery takeoff from the popliteal vessel just proximal to the interosseous membrane. Then 1 to 2 cm distally the peroneal artery takes off laterally from the posterior tibial artery while the posterior tibial artery continues medially. An arteriogram can provide a preoperative map of these three vessels and their relationship to each other. However, it is still extremely important to be certain as to the vascular anatomy in situ at the time of dissection before any major vessels are divided or the flap is harvested. For this reason, we do not routinely obtain an arteriogram in the normal leg from which a free fibula flap is to be harvested, especially in the younger patient.

The full length of the incision is generally not made until the trifurcation in the proximal leg and the popliteal fossa are readily identified. Once the takeoff of the peroneal artery is identified, one can then estimate the length of pedicle that is available. This will determine the level at which the proximal fibula should be divided. The distal division level is then determined by the length of fibula that is needed at the recipient site.

The anterior incision is determined by the width of the skin island that is desired. The skin island is elevated from anterior to lateral just superficial to the anterior compartment muscles and peroneal muscles until the lateral fibula border is reached. Here the peroneal muscles can be stripped off of the anterior border of the fibula, leaving little or no muscle attached to the fibula in this position (Figure 14.7). Alternatively, the incision can continue down through the lateral peroneal muscles, leaving a cuff of peroneal musculature on the fibula anteriorly. In either event, the septum between the peroneal muscles and the soleus muscles should not be entered, as this is the septum which provides septocutaneous perforators to the overlying skin island. Medially, the anterior tibial vessels, which lie deep in the anterior compartment on the interosseous septum, should also be identified and protected. The superficial peroneal nerve is often sacrificed if the peroneal musculature is harvested with the flap, since this nerve runs superficially through this musculature and eventually subcutaneously.

Division of the fibula should not be within 6 cm of the proximal fibula head or 6 to 8 cm of the distal fibula so as not to interfere with either knee or ankle joint function. However, if further length is taken toward the distal fibula, the remaining segment of fibula should be fixed to the tibia using a cortical screw. The fibula is divided proximally and distally at the desired length using a Gigli saw prior to the dissection of the posterior compartment. At this point in the dissection, the flap is free in its bed with the peroneal vessels isolated. It is completely detached from the remain-

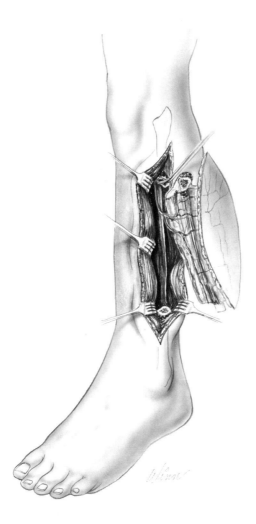

Figure 14.7.   Elevation of free fibula flap.

ing soleus muscle laterally and the peroneal muscles and anterior compartment medially. The interosseous membrane is divided with the scissors.

Retracting this entire flap laterally allows the continuation of the peroneal vessels to be seen just deep to the distally divided fibula. These vessels are ligated and divided. Intramuscular dissection is then performed within the flexor hallucis longus and the tibialis posterior muscle, leaving a cuff of 1 to 2 cm of each of these muscles on the posterior fibula. This is to avoid injury to the peroneal pedicle, which runs along the posteromedial border of the fibula, providing periosteal perforators as well as septo-cutaneous perforators. The flap is now freed as an island (Figure 14.8). The tourniquet is released and hemostasis is achieved. It is important to obtain hemostasis rapidly so that as much swelling as possible can be avoided. This will assist in direct skin closure.

There are several important elements in preparation of the recipient site. First, the medullary cavity of the tibia, both proximal and distal, must be large enough to accept the free fibula flap. Curetting or reaming of the medullary cavity may be necessary. Secondly, the surrounding bed in the recipient leg should be adequately debrided so that the bed will accept the

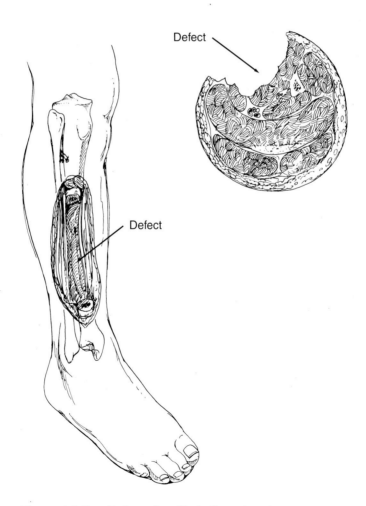

Figure 14.8. Defect after fibula flap elevation.

muscle bulk of the free fibula flap. The elevation technique in raising the free fibula flap can minimize the surrounding muscle, but there is always a cuff of soleus, posterior tibialis, and flexor hallucis longus which will bring some bulk to the wound. This should be anticipated.

The pedicle choice in terms of size and location is critical in the success of this flap and the survival of the overlying skin island. The skin island and the pedicle basically lie at 180° from each other on the free fibula flap. At the recipient site it is difficult to alter this relationship greatly without compromising the delicate septocutaneous vessels to the overlying skin island. The peroneal vessels of the flap therefore generally exit the receiving tibial bed either posteromedially or posterolaterally. The preferred location is posteromedially, since that is where the posterior tibial vessels are located (Figure 14.9). These make excellent donor vessels if they are available, because they are of good size and in the proper location. If a posterior tibial cortex is present, an exit hole of adequate size can be made to provide an outlet for the peroneal vessels to extend from the inset flap to the posterior tibial vessels.

The fibula is then inset within the medullary cavity of the tibia while simultaneously orienting the peroneal vessels to be in proximity to the posterior tibial vessels without tension on either the peroneal vessels or the overlying skin island. The bone can then be stabilized proximally and distally with a lag screw, and additional bone graft is usually placed around the proximal and distal ends of the fibula. Revascularization follows, generally using an end-to-side technique for the arterial anastomosis.

External fixation provides an excellent protective device during the early days and weeks after free fibula transfer. Monitoring the flap is done using the parameters as described for the scapular free flap. In addition, a bone scan may be obtained within the first week after free fibula transfer to document blood flow into the flap. If the bone scan is done more than a week after transfer, peripheral bony revascularization may be confused with primary revascularization through microvascular reanastomosis. The external fixator, however, may be looked upon as a two-edged sword as the patient enters the 2- to 6-month postoperative period. Activity is in-

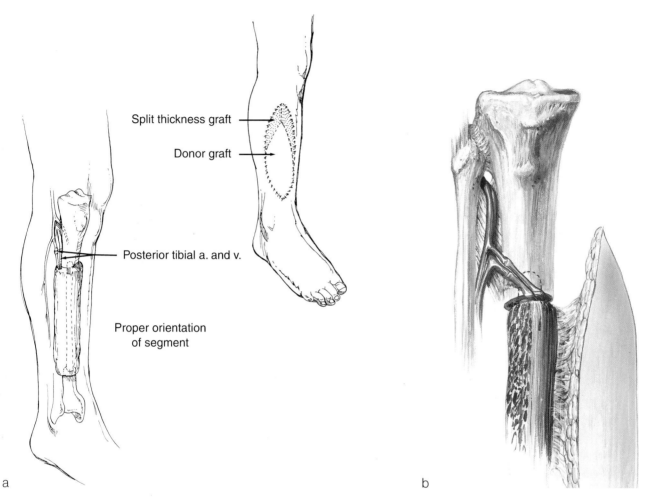

Split thickness graft

Donor graft

Posterior tibial a. and v.

Proper orientation
of segment

a

b

Figure 14.9. Proper orientation of fibular flap: (a) Segment positioned properly. (b) Improper orientation of flap vessels.

creased and some weight-bearing is allowed with the external fixator in place. However, during the period from 4 to 6 months some weight-bearing with stress is allowed on the reconstructive site. This aids in strengthening and thickening of the free bone transfer. Gradually, increasing stress can be accomplished using walking casts as substitutes for the external fixator. However, it should be remembered that complete healing of both proximal and distal bony anastomotic sites may take from 8 to 12 months, depending on the age of the patient and the status of the wound.

Discussion

The free fibular flap has been refined significantly over the last 15 years from a bulky, rather unwieldy flap with a large overlying skin island to one that only carries that which is needed for the wound.[19-21] Refinement in flap harvest is due to a more precise knowledge of the blood supply to the periosteum of the fibula and to the overlying skin island.[22] This has made the free fibular transfer a safer flap without the unnecessary bulk of surrounding muscles. Bulkiness of the surrounding musculature can be a decided liability if this contributes to compression upon the peroneal blood supply after the fibula is placed within its restricted space at the recipient site.

The free fibula remains the leading choice for replacement of a missing segment of tibia greater than 6 cm. The Ilizarov technique has proven successful in defects up to 12 cm. However, the lengthy period (12 months) needed for bone transport diminished the attraction of this technique to many patients. For this reason, patients with longer segments of missing bone (>6 cm) will continue to turn to free vascularized bony transfer for treatment.

Other possible sites for consideration include the free scapular bone flap and the free iliac crest flap. Although these flaps do provide very strong cortical bone essential for replacement to the tibia, they each have their own drawbacks. The free iliac crest bone is curved and does not fit as neatly within the tibial bed in most cases. The lateral border of the scapular free flap, while straight, does not provide the same density of bone as is found with the fibula. All of these donor sites have similar morbidity from pain, scarring, and loss of function.

Donor site disability due to the free fibula harvest is a concern when one considers the muscle units that are divided and the amount of bone that is removed. However, an anatomical closure of the donor site with adequate closed-suction drainage systems almost invariably leads to an uncomplicated wound closure with little or no debility in that extremity.[18] Excessive fibula harvest, either proximally or distally, should be avoided, since this can increase the morbidity of the harvest.

Significant retraction injury to the lateral peroneal nerve can also be avoided, since this nerve is visible early in the dissection process. However, injury to this nerve can lead to foot drop and paresthesias of the anterior distal leg or foot, which is disconcerting and can be avoided.[17]

Healing is prolonged, as with any significant bony injury, but a successful outcome can be expected with appropriate postoperative protection and rehabilitation. Resection of nonunions proximally or distally followed by bone grafting may be necessary in a small percentage of cases, but this is not frequent. Furthermore, fracture of the transferred fibula in the mid-shaft, as noted in this case, can occur if adequate protection of the fibula is not provided for 8 to 12 months postoperatively or until thickening of the fibula secondary to stress can be documented by radiography.

ROUNDTABLE DISCUSSION

DR. ELLIOTT

The free fibula was chosen in this patient primarily because he had a defect greater than 6 cm in the distal tibia. Numerous studies indicate that greater than 6 cm of bony loss requires more than simple bone grafting. The Ilizarov bone transport technique offers new options in this area of reconstruction, but transport of greater than 6 cm is still on the fringes of acceptability. The vascularized bone flap is more successful in establishing union.

DR. ZUBOWICZ

My approach to the open bony wound is as follows: first, clean the wound; second, close the wound; and third, deal with the bony situation. In general, management of the bone is the responsibility of the orthopedic surgeon, not the plastic surgeon. We generally respond to their request for vascularized bone. But it is our responsibility to provide them with the environment to get the bone to heal. I have no problem at all with first debriding the wound and leaving it open for whatever period of time it takes, even if it takes weeks, until the wound gets stabilized. Then it can be closed, of course making use of the external fixation device which is prevalent now. At some time later—even if it is many months later—when the inflammation has subsided, the bony problem can be addressed. If the wound is clean and the orthopedic surgeon is convinced that vascularized bone is needed, then I think you can skip the middle step, as was done in this particular case, and reconstruct the bone and soft tissue concurrently. But I would chastise anyone who would try to skip the middle step as a way of cutting corners.

DR. GROTTING

First, I want to point out that it is extremely advantageous if one can maintain a space between the injured ends of the tibia in which the fibula will eventually be placed. One of the ways this can be done is with placement of methylmethacrylate antibiotic beads in the cavity simply to maintain the space there for your eventual bone transfer. Second, with regard to specifics of the free fibula transfer, it should be pointed out that after 6 to 8 hours of operating, it is often not possible to close the soft tissues over the transferred fibula. For this reason, it is very nice to have a skin island with the transferred fibula. Admittedly, there are only two or three septocutaneous vessels that perfuse the overlying skin island at either end of the skin island. However, our practice has been to include a long ellipse of skin over the entire length of fibula that is going to be transferred and carry the incision down, taking the peroneal muscles off the posterolateral intermuscular septum. We do the same thing with the soleus. This sacrifices a minimal amount of muscle at the donor site and leaves less muscle on the flap itself. This has been particularly advantageous in mandibular reconstruction, where less muscle bulk is needed. This also preserves the septocutaneous vessels that come off the peroneal vessels and has improved the reliability of the skin island. Third, I feel that to achieve proper osteosynthesis, the tibial canal should be reamed and the fibula inserted into the tibia after periosteum has been stripped off each end of the fibula, so as to preserve those crucial vessels to the skin island of the free fibula flap.

DR. STAHL

I would like to make three points. First, while my bias leads me to agree with the 6-cm division line between vascularized and nonvascularized bone grafts, I think this is based on relatively older data and needs to be proven again. This is especially true in view of the Ilizarov technique and its increasingly widespread use. Second, I would also warn against using the fibula from the injured leg, since this fibula can be very important in the stability of the leg with the fracture. Third, with regard to the specifics of harvesting the flap, I prefer to do osteotomies very early on in the elevation of the flap. The pedicle is then dissected retrogradely as opposed to starting in the popliteal fossa and encircling the vessels initially.

DR. TOTH

Preoperative preparation is essential to the achievement of an efficiently executed procedure. You should make sure that your external fixation pins have been moved if they are going to be in the way. Decisions with regard to the external fixation device should be made preoperatively so that changes will not be made during the procedure. The wound must be adequately debrided prior to your free bone transfer so that all efforts can be focused upon the safe execution of a free bone transfer without wasting large amounts of time in changing hardware or additional debridement.

DR. MOSES

The fibula is a good choice because it is straight compared to the other options for vascularized bone, the pelvis or the scapula. The bad news is that the fibula is too thin. Its dimensions allow it to be fitted into the tibial medullary cavity, but it is thinner than the tibia and therefore requires an extended period of protection against full weight-bearing, to avoid fracturing before the bone hypertrophies, as demonstrated in this case.

DR. ELLIOTT

How long is "extended?" I agree with you that fractures can be seen in the mid-shaft of the transplanted fibula, but this is part and parcel of tibia reconstruction and attests to the prolonged period of 6 to 9 months of protection with gradual weight-bearing.

DR. MOSES

I agree that bony hypertrophy is in response to stress and that this stress should be gradually increased while following the bony hypertrophy with frequent radiographs and adjusting the cast or splint.

DR. TOTH

I would like to again emphasize the importance of not harvesting the ipsilateral fibula, which would further disrupt the potential strength and integrity of the leg.

DR. ZUBOWICZ

While I agree that the ipsilateral fibula cannot be routinely harvested, we have done this before at the request of the orthopedic surgeon. It can be done and occasionally is the best choice. However, usually the ipsilateral fibula is in the zone of surgery and cannot be used.

DR. MOSES

With regard to the ipsilateral fibula, I think the decision is in large part dependent on vascularity. Many patients with such severe trauma have had injury to one or two of the three main vessels of the leg. In that case, harvesting the fibula with the intentional sacrifice of peroneal vessels might be extremely detrimental to the vascularity of the injured leg.

DR. ELLIOTT

I have touched on monitoring in Chapter 13. In this case, the skin island may provide an ability to monitor, but we don't always transfer the skin island because of bulk problems. The bone viability can be monitored by bone scanning, but that has to be done early, within the first 1 to 2 days, and then it cannot be repeated as often as one might like for monitoring purposes. We do try to place the pedicle so that it can be followed with a Doppler probe or directly inspected through a skin graft if that is practical. Inspection of the muscle through a skin graft is another choice, but this depends greatly on the inspector's experience. Obviously, the totally buried flap cannot be monitored in any of these ways and has to be monitored expectantly.

DR. ZUBOWICZ

If I could summarize the choices for vascularized bone, considering all the carpentry problems and donor morbidity problems, it is my impression that the vascularized fibula stands far above all the possible donor choices.

REFERENCES

1. Ilizarov GA. The tension-stress effect on the genesis and growth of tissues. Part I. Clin Orthop Rel Res 1989;238:249.

2. Ilizarov GA. The tension-stress effect on the genesis and growth of tissues. Part II. Clin Orthop Rel Res 1989;239:263.

3. Cierny G III, Zorn KE. Bony reconstruction in the lower extremity. Clin Plast Surg 1992;19:905.

4. Weiland AJ, Moore JR, Daniel RK. Vascularized bone autografts: experience with 41 cases. Clin Orthop 1983;174:87.

5. Taylor GI. The current status of free vascularized bone grafts. Clin Plast Surg 1983;10:185.

6. Byrd HS, Spicer TE, Cierny G III. Management of open tibial fractures. Plast Reconstr Surg 1985;76:719.

7. Weiland AJ, Daniel RK. Microvascular anastomoses for bone grafts in the treatment of massive defects in bone. J Bone Joint Surg 1979;61A:98.

8. Gilbert A. Free transfer of the fibular shaft. Int J Microsurg 1979;1:1.

9. Hidalgo DA. Aesthetic improvements in free-flap mandible reconstruction. Plast Reconstr Surg 1991;88:575.

INDEX